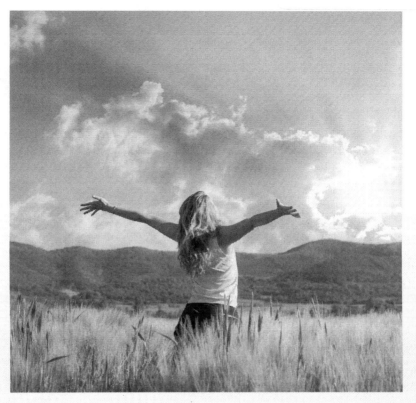

The Stress Eating Solution

EMOTIONAL BRAIN TRAINING

Laurel Mellin, PhD

Emotional Brain Training (EBT) is a science-based program of emotional neuroplasticity in which people use simple tools to raise their brain's set point for optimal well-being. As with any skills training program, EBT is not without risk and may be unsafe or ineffective for some people. If you have any psychological or medical problems, consult with your physician and other health professionals before beginning this program. EBT is not medical care, but skills training that can be used in support of improved preventive and therapeutic healthcare outcomes. Using the program with the training and support of a Certified EBT Provider is recommended. The outcomes associated with self-study use of EBT are not known. The author, The Solution Foundation (a non-profit corporation), and EBT, Inc. (a California corporation) disclaim all liability for any adverse effects that may result from the use or application of the information contained in this book. The characters discussed in this publication are composites of several individuals and the names of all individuals have been changed to maintain anonymity. Certified EBT Providers may be licensed or registered health professionals. However, they facilitate EBT services outside of their license(s). All providers complete both personal and professional training in the method. To learn more about certification training in EBT, visit ebtbook.com/stresseating. For a complete list of EBT resources, see "Your EBT Experience" on page 277. If you have questions about the EBT program, please email your inquiry to support@ebt.org. Previously-published books on the tools are no longer reflective of the latest advances in neuroscience. We recommend that you use the techniques described in the books by this author that were published in 2019 or later.

Editors: Frannie Wilson and Michele Welling. InDesign production: Jamie Holecek. Graphics design: Steven Isakson. Graphics consultant: Jami Spittler. Production: Michael McClure. Technology: Dev Singh and Andrea Singh. Technology design: Joe Mellin. Creative adviser: Walt Rose. Manager: Kelly McGrath. Cover photography: Jamie Rain.

ISBN: 978-0-9864107-7-2
Author: Laurel Mellin, PhD
Published by: EBT Books,
a division of EBT, Inc.
101 Larkspur Landing Circle, Suite 327, Larkspur, CA 94939
WEBSITE: www.ebt.org
E-MAIL: support@ebt.org

Also by Laurel Mellin

The Stress Overload Solution
Wired for Joy
Spiral Up!
The Pathway
The Solution
Shapedown
3-Day Solution Plan

For Walt

Contents

Release Weight

Celebrate Your Joy

Introduction

Imagine yourself awakening in the morning and realizing that you only have one job for the day. You are going to connect to the deepest part of yourself and process your emotions with symphonic precision and return to your joy. Your job is to create joy in your life!

Sure, you had lists of things to do, people to see, and challenges to meet, but that's only what the outside world could see. Internally, privately, and magically, you were working busily away at a far more important task. You were using each moment to process your emotions, strengthening your wires that made you naturally joyful. As the emotion joy is the sign that your entire being is at its best, wiring your brain for joy was a simple, effective solution to life.

As your brain developed the joy habit, food and weight stopped being issues in your life. You found more peace and confidence within. When you noticed that you were stressed, you would smile to yourself and say, "That's not a problem. I'm in pre-joy mode. I just need to process those emotions and I'll return to my joy."

When you got the urge to eat in the evening, you took out your app, used the tools, and the hunger faded. Then you started releasing weight, and it wasn't that hard! You realized that all along the problem had not been you. It was that you needed more joy in your life. They joy chemicals calm the appetite and bring you the safety, love, comfort, and pleasure you need – without abusing food, obsessing about food, or even thinking about food!

The purpose of this book is to help you become wired for joy. It's based on the tools of emotional brain training (EBT) and the Brain Based Health approach to life. It's to use the brain for its highest and best purpose – to process our emotions. As you process your emotions, wires that trigger stress eating change. They transform into wires that promote healthy eating.

As the wires change, you'll notice you are eating healthier with little or no effort. You'll stop seeing overeating as a behavior. It's just the tail end of a wire in the brain that stored an emotional response, an expectation of what to do, and a drive to engage in a specific action. Overeating is actually a three-step process.

Step 1. Something triggers us – and a wire is activated

The strings of neurons, or wires, that are stored in our emotional brain control most of our responses in life. Right now, if you are feeling good and are free of food cravings, you're probably running a highly effective wire. We call it a Joy Circuit. However, we all have another kind of circuit, a Stress Circuit, and if a sensation, emotion, thought, or behavior happens to trigger one of your Stress Circuits; specifically, one that triggers overeating, every cell, organ, and organ system in your body will be affected.

Step 2. That wire causes cascades of stress chemicals

If your brain activates a Stress Circuit, including the specific circuit that triggers your overeating, you will experience a chemical effect. That's because the Stress Circuit activates the brain's Stress Triangle. This triangle is comprised of three structures that control our body chemistry. They are the amygdala ("stress center"), nucleus accumbens ("reward center") and the hypothalamus ("appetite center"). Robert Lustig and Michele Mietus-Snyder first recognized this triangle, stating that the drives from these three centers make overeating and weight gain almost inevitable. Once activated, these three centers spew chemical surges, causing imbalances that make us hungry, lethargic, depressed, and overweight.

Joy Circuits

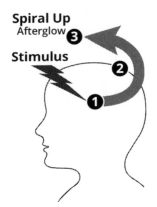

Spiral Up
Afterglow ❸

Stimulus

❶ Accurate Emotions
A stimulus enters the brain
and activates balanced feelings.

❷ Reasonable Expectations
An accurate message guides us
(e.g., I get my safety from inside me).

❸ Effective Response
We respond in an adaptive way
(e.g., We eat healthy).

Step 3. We stress eat! The chemicals make us do it!

What do we do? We do what that wire tells us to do. We overeat! The amygdala activates a Stress Circuit, and the reward center makes us crave highly palatable foods that add to our stress. Our stress-activated chemicals control us, causing cravings (high dopamine), hunger (ghrelin and insulin), and over time, depression (low serotonin), and weight gain (leptin). The hypothalamus causes us to feel lethargic. What do we do to get our energy back? We overeat! The Stress Triangle spins out of control, and we become stuck in the stress eating cycle. The solution? Break free of that stress eating cycle!

Stress Circuits

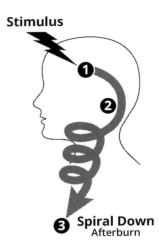

Stimulus

❸ Spiral Down
Afterburn

❶ Inaccurate Emotions
A stimulus enters the brain and activates
cravings, overreactions, or shutdowns.

❷ Unreasonable Expectations
An inaccurate message drives us
(e.g., I get my safety from eating sweets).

❸ Ineffective Response
We respond in a maladaptive way
(e.g., We overeat).

Why not go to the root cause of the problem?

If the problem is that Stress Circuits activate chemicals that cause cravings, lethargy, depression, and weight gain, why not shut off that circuit and, in its place, activate a Joy Circuit, that makes us sensible about food? The EBT tool that guides us along our resiliency pathway delivers the oddest thing – a successful and quick emotional meltdown.

We jumpstart our journey from stress to joy by stating what we're stressed about since even briefly articulating what bothers us reduces our stress. Then we artfully express anger, sadness, fear, and guilt, which releases those pent-up suppressed emotions, and triggers something wonderful: an unexpected surge of positive emotions. When you first give this technique a try, it can be a bit astonishing. A few moments before, food and life looked drastically different. The "I gotta have it" drive to eat sugary, fatty processed foods has vanished, and you feel emotionally lighter! You might even wonder, "What just happened?" You have used your brain's resiliency pathway. That's the power of that hidden pathway. Its effects can seem magical!

Your transition to using emotions in rather amazing ways and thinking in terms of wires, not issues or problems, takes time. To get off to a great start with using this brain-based method, take these three steps:

Step 1. Stop all food judgments

The emotional brain or "stress brain" can't stand to be judged or shamed. This invites an instant triggering of one of our Stress Circuits. Until the last 10 years, we didn't know that the root cause of overeating was Stress Circuits and had no idea that we had a resiliency pathway, much less tools to give us new power to use it! The first step in transitioning to brain-based healthcare is to stop judging your eating, your weight, and yourself!

Prepare for Success
Step 1. Stop all food judgments.
Step 2. Use clear, brain-based language about stress eating.
Step 3. Have fun using the tools!

Step 2. Use clear, brain-based language about stress eating

Go ahead and start talking to other people about your eating and weight, but use brain-based concepts and language. That will nudge your unconscious mind to shift to the new paradigm.

I told my daughter that I am working on the wire that makes me want to binge on cookies. She had no idea what I was talking about, but in time it will sink in. I want her to know she has the power to change her habits but needs to address the root cause: a pathway in her brain.

My buddy is a drinker. He has a drinking wire, and my wire is overeating. We both have wires to work on, and I think my food wire is at least as strong as his drinking wire.

My best friend and I ate our way through our divorces, and when we get together, she talks about doing things like going on a fast together. I tell her that I am dealing with my food wire. My project is to short-circuit that wire, to eat healthy naturally. The more I talk about wires, the more powerful and excited I feel. This could be fun.

Step 3. Have fun using the tools!

Most healing methods are pretty serious. Whether we use cognitive methods, insight-oriented psychotherapy, or diet plans, there isn't a lot of joy and merriment or even aha moments. EBT is full of fun times.

For instance, a few months ago, I was in the lobby of the San Francisco Hyatt Regency. Having just delivered a presentation on EBT at an obesity medicine conference, I was relaxing, relieved to be done. I noticed a physician with a conference badge on her jacket hurrying along the nearby hallway. She was raising an oversized candy bar to her mouth, about to take a bite.

Our eyes met, and at first, she blanched, but then we both smiled, musing at the irony of the experience. An obesity doctor who had just listened to my talk was about to succumb to stress eating!

I called out to her half-jokingly, "Do you want to give EBT a try? It only takes a couple of minutes!"

She smiled, blinked twice, and then nodded eagerly. She came right over, sat down next to me, and I began guiding her through one of the EBT tools. About three minutes later, her face brightened. That meant that the tool had worked. She was at Brain State 1, optimal connection, which shuts off the chemicals that drive cravings, hunger, lethargy, and weight gain.

The woman widened her eyes. She laughed, placing both hands over her mouth. She said, "Oh my gosh. It actually works!"

Then she looked down at the candy bar on her lap. She winced and told me, "A few minutes ago, all I could think about was this candy. I craved it. I HAD to have it. Now, it looks completely . . . disgusting to me! All those preservatives, the corn syrup, and those fake ingredients!"

A moment later she dashed back toward the lecture hall, and before disappearing into the crowd, she darted over to a nearby receptacle – and tossed the candy bar into the trash.

Enjoy exploring your unconscious mind

To shut off a Stress Circuit, we must break it open so it reveals hidden emotions and expectations. We bring to our awareness the messages that have been stored away in our unconscious mind. When the offending wire (such as the stress eating circuit) is activated, the reason we have been overeating becomes clear to us. Sometimes, in what we call a "travel back" we can even re-experience the moment that the circuit was encoded. That happened to me as I rewired my stress eating wire.

One day I was using the tools when I was so angry at myself for craving sugar and being completely out of control of my eating. All of a sudden, my mind flashed on the moment when my stress eating wire was encoded. I was 11 years old, and had come home from school after a really hard day. One girl, Janet, was bullying me, and I had just run for 6th grade vice president and lost miserably. The school secretary posted the vote count on the office bulletin board for everyone to see. Next to my name was my vote count: two, and one was my own vote from myself!

After dropping my school books on the kitchen table, I spotted a rectangular package of cinnamon rolls with white swirls of icing on the counter. A light in my brain turned on, and I went for them. I ate three big ones and encoded my food wire, which stayed stuck in my brain for over 20 years, triggering sugar binges, overeating, and a strong drive to use food as a love substitute. I had no idea then that it was just a wire – one that I would later rewire. However, from that experience of discovering the wire, I stopped judging myself about my sugar cravings and food binges and felt more peace and power from within. The sacred nature of that moment of recognition continues to nourish and deepen my love for myself, and, ultimately, it is that loving connection within that shuts off overeating, and activates the desire to eat healthy.

We need a new, brain-based approach

We have tried so hard to stop overeating by using traditional approaches. They were all developed 50 to 100 years ago, before 1990 when the decade of the brain ushered in new approaches based on neuroplasticity. We have tried! We have stapled our stomachs, debated diets, instituted legislation against sodas, displayed calorie counts on menus, and cleaned up areas lacking access to healthy food. Yet despite these massive efforts to promote healthy eating habits, the U.S. daily consumption averaged 2,481 calories per person in 2010, up 23 percent from energy intake in 1970. Our vegetable and fruit intake is down 14 percent since 1970. Comfort food intake (refined carbohydrates and fats) makes up 60 percent of our calories.

Currently, according to government statistics, 70 percent of Americans meet the criteria for overweight, and 40 percent meet the criteria for obesity. The cost of obesity, from diminished life expectancy and lost income tallies up to $8,365 for women and $6,518 for men per person annually. The national estimated annual healthcare cost of weight-related illness is $190 billion, amounting to about 21 percent of healthcare expenditures in the United States. Yet we continue using failed approaches rather than going to the root cause of the problem and rewiring the drive to overeat.

With all this emphasis on what we eat and no simple system for categorizing our stress eating style or changing the wiring that activates it, our relationship with food has suffered, too. More and more of us are stressed about what we eat. Nearly 80 percent of women and almost 70 percent of men in the U.S. report guilt about food, and about half of all adults report overeating enough in the last month to have a food hangover. Eating disorders throughout the world are on the rise, with 70 million people suffering from binge eating disorder. Neuroscience has advanced so dramatically, that there is no reason for us to suffer like this. It's time to apply brain science to overeating and overweight so that we can experience optimal well-being – and more joy in our lives!

The 6 pioneers of EBT for stress eating

In developing this method, my colleagues and I closely adhered to the emerging sciences of neuroplasticity and neurophysiology. For this EBT stress eating program, we drew most heavily upon the work of these six scientific pioneers:

Pioneer #1: Michael Merzenich, PhD – The father of neuroplasticity

Neuroscientist Michael Merzenich discovered that the brain is soft-wired, and proposed that the new science of brain plasticity can change our lives. His contributions range from being on the team that developed the cochlear implant for hearing loss to rewiring the brains of children, whether it is to overcome learning problems or to heal from trauma. Through his research in experience-dependent learning with non-human primates, he demonstrated that neuroplasticity remains through adulthood. Dr. Merzenich is a professor emeritus at UCSF and has contributed to more than 230 scientific articles. As a co-founder and Chief Scientific Officer of Posit Science, Dr. Merzenich heads the company's science team. He holds nearly 100 patents and spearheaded brain training as a new field in healthcare.

Pioneer #2: Igor Mitrovic, MD – The scientific director

Neuroscientist and physiologist Igor Mitrovic began using the method personally in 2004, and, realizing that the book he was reading on the method was authored by another UCSF professor, contacted me, and the rest is history. As Dr. Mitrovic used the method, he sought to explain why it worked. He could see that it did, but as a scientist, he sought to identify its biologic basis. He conceptualized brain wires as either effective ("homeostatic") or ineffective ("allostatic"). By defining these wires, they became entities to target and rewire. In collaboration with Lynda Frassetto, MD, Lindsey Fish, MD, and me, he conceived of EBT as a new paradigm in healthcare. Instead of treating the symptoms of these stress wires, we could go to the source and change the wiring itself.

Pioneer #3: Robert Lustig, MD – The stress triangle originator

You may know of UCSF professor and endocrinologist Robert Lustig for his work with obesity and sugar, as well as addiction. His books, *Fat Chance* and *The Hacking of the American Mind* are great reading and background for this book. With colleague Michele Mietus-Snyder, a preventive cardiologist at the Children's National Health System, Dr. Lustig conceptualized the Stress Triangle (Limbic Triangle) in the emotional brain, three brain structures – the stress, appetite, and reward centers – that cause overeating and weight gain. This is the triangle we seek to tame by using the EBT tools.

Pioneer #4: Mary Dallman, PhD – The comfort eating researcher

Another UCSF professor, Mary Dallman, a neurophysiologist, discovered the relationship between overeating and stress. In fact, she showed that when we consume sugary, fatty foods, the brain's stress center ("amygdala") calms down. For the moment, our stress eases. The stress hormone ("cortisol") cascade that feeds the Stress Triangle quiets down. That temporary "honeymoon" of calm is followed by the widespread amplification of stress, hunger, and cravings that causes weight gain and deposition of belly fat. The dopamine highs caused by sugar result in the draining of serotonin, so we are not only hungry and heavy, but depressed and sick.

Pioneer #5: Elizabeth Phelps, PhD – The emotional rewiring scientist

Elizabeth Phelps, PhD, professor of neuroscience at Harvard University, conducted ground-breaking research that helps us understand more about how we can change our wiring. In her collaborations with Joseph LeDoux, Director of New York University's Emotional Brain Institute, she showed that these circuits are highly plastic, however, rewiring them requires an emotional spark – a stress activation. The EBT tools deliver that stress activation, whereas traditional methods do not include that essential spark.

Pioneer #6: Bruce McEwen, PhD – The chief of stress research

The last of the pioneers is Bruce McEwen from Rockefeller University. His work on emotional plasticity theory is at the heart of EBT, explaining the persistence of eating and weight problems as symptoms of the cumulative effect of stress on the brain (allostatic load). With repeated episodes of psychological stress, and the additional stress from many sources, including eating sugary, fatty foods, and carrying extra weight, our stress "buzzer" becomes stuck on. This means that the Stress Triangle is chronically activated so even if we get a handle on healthy eating or weight loss, its biochemical surges (cortisol, insulin, ghrelin, leptin, and dopamine) are likely to cause rebound of overeating and overweight. Whom have we blamed for that? We have blamed ourselves, but no longer. The pathway to lasting improvements in eating and weight loss based on Dr. McEwen's contributions is reducing stress overload and raising our brain's set point.

If it's not fun, it's not EBT

I hope you find this book both fun and life-changing. You may never have started a healthy eating and weight program that told you your job is to create joy in your life, but joy is not optional. The brain insists that we feel rewarded, and if we do not deliver to it an abundance of natural pleasures, it finds artificial ones. Stress and artificial rewards can reduce the brain's capacity to feel good, amplifying our drive to use artificial rewards just to feel normal. In fact, about 30 percent of us are reward insufficient, with a low number of dopamine receptors, and most of the rest of us have a mild version of that. Radical joy becomes our needed defense against the addictive drives to overeat.

The joy of emotional connection

The brain's ultimate natural pleasure is emotional connection. Each moment of warm connection with another person offers a surge of oxytocin, the natural appetite suppressant. Add to that the observation that the emotional brain changes best when we connect with others, and our emphasis on community makes perfect sense. You can create your own community with family and friends who are reading this book and/or join the EBT Community for ready-made private connections and small groups. Just visit ebt.org to join. Use the coupon code: stresseating to receive a discount on our Online PLUS membership.

Honoring our amazing power

As you learn these tools, you may become more aware of the power of your emotions. You might find that you become more vibrant and emotionally alive – sometimes silly and playful, sometimes pensive, other times full of passion!

The EBT method makes it safe to be fully alive to your feelings. You can lean into your feelings and enjoy having a successful emotional meltdown, as you know those few moments of emotional intensity can be life-changing! You might wonder why everyone doesn't know about EBT! All of it is based on neuroscience, and the tools give you a way to use your own emotional brain to its best effect. You always had this brain, the product of evolution and a miracle in its own way. All you ever needed were a few tools to use it well. You are now on the pathway to getting them. Thank you for your interest in EBT, and I hope you find this course opens doors in your mind, and gives you a new level of love for yourself, for others, and for life!

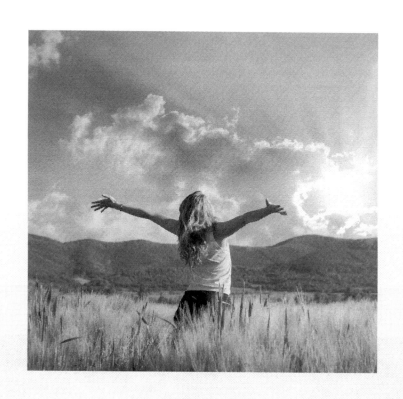

Welcome

The Power of Joy

The pathway in your brain that moves you from stress to joy may be your most valuable asset! It enables you to dip down into stress, give yourself an emotional cleanse, then spiral you back to a state of well-being. The Stress Triangle stops spinning and eating healthy and releasing extra weight become remarkably easy. Yes, easy!

The power of joy is astonishing. According to neuroscientist Anastasio Damasio, joy signifies the smooth workings of the operations of life. When we are in the "joy state," the chemical and electrical surges that activate cravings, hunger, depression, lethargy, and weight gain quiet down.

The EBT strategy to end overeating skips calorie counting and instead, counts moments of natural pleasure – Joy Points! Rather than calculating your caloric needs, you appraise how many moments of joy you require to stop wanting extra food. By training the brain to deliver that much joy, healthy eating and lasting weight loss can naturally follow.

Tonight, at dinner I ate half what I normally do. I was full and satisfied on less food. How did that happen?

Joy is a Brain State

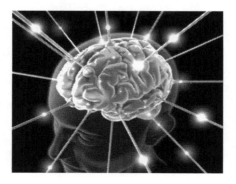

1

My pants are loose. I'm not sure why. I've been taking care of my body, but I'm not on a diet. My body seems to want to release weight.

This is an exciting and fun course. Each day for 30 days you will learn one tool for creating joy in your life, then you will take another 30 days to make solid four new wires in your brain.

The next step? Honor your brain's natural desire for the seven rewards of a purposeful life – Sanctuary, Authenticity, Vibrancy, Integrity, Intimacy, Spirituality, and Freedom. Training your inner life to access these rewards raises your set point for profound and lasting changes in your life.

The EBT Program

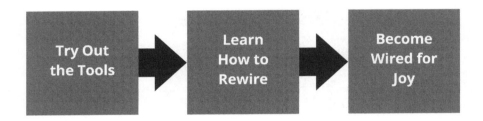

Step 1: Try Out the Tools
Begin by trying out the tools. The first few days of this challenge are aimed at helping you learn how to use the tools to get from stress to joy. Discover that you can create joy in your life. It's just a skill! Instead of trying to figure out how to feel better, reach for the tools and switch off stress and activate joy. Savor these first experiences in discovering the amazing powers of your brain!

Step 2: Learn How to Rewire
After learning how to switch the brain from stress to joy, learn how to rewire. Start with rewiring the drive to overeat and boost the new wiring's strength by rewiring a stuck mood, a challenging relationship pattern, and a leftover harmful attitude toward your body. Along the way, shape your lifestyle to bring you far more natural pleasure and vibrant living. Take time after that ("the second 30 days") to continue using these tools, giving your brain time to reorganize itself around a higher level of functioning ("higher set point"). When you feel ready for more, go on to Step 3.

Step 3: Become Wired for Joy
Once food and weight are no longer issues in your life, your unconscious mind will hunger for you to emotionally evolve. You will sense that there is no going back. You have already changed so much, why stop now? Whereas previously you came to EBT to solve a problem, now your interest naturally turns to accessing more of the rewards of a purposeful life: Sanctuary, Authenticity, Vibrancy, Integrity, Intimacy, Spirituality, and Freedom. You move into Advanced EBT, starting with the first advanced course – *Sanctuary: Peace and power from within.*

This last phase of the training is the most important. You will be encoding circuits in your brain that create sturdy emotional pathways that move you through stress and its attendant self-doubt, shame, blame, disgust, and paralysis to a sense of safety from within, profound love, healthy comforts, and natural pleasure. The circuits that promote resilience will land you squarely into a world of purpose. The drive for artificial "hedonic" rewards, which so often deranges the elegance of our physiology, fades as we train our brain for the natural "eudonic" rewards of life.

After using the tools in this book to clear away circuits that block your joy, you can continue to use the tools to create a more secure connection with yourself. By doing so, you encode in your wiring the virtues of life that will hold you through any loss or challenge. What arises is a spiritual sufficiency that brings you self-reliance and freedom to do what you came to Earth to do. Imagine, it all began because you had a desire to stop overeating!

When we step through the portal of the unconscious mind in pursuit of what we want, more often than not the universe or something greater than ourselves gives us precisely what we most need. It often arrives not in small measure, but in abundance.

How Does It Work?

Until the last decade, it was thought that our tangle of brain wires, or circuits, could not be changed. Or, if we could possibly change them, it was thought to require medications, surgeries, devices, psychotherapy, or something else that was not within our complete control.

Now we know differently. We can train our brain – remodel it based on experience. The brain constantly reorganizes itself, updating our wiring. The very wires that impact our health and happiness the most are highly plastic. If we use emotional tools and focused attention, we can alter our own wiring! We can spot a problem that bothers us, use simple emotional tools, and weaken the wire causing the problem. If we want to encode a new and better wire, we can do that, too. This is a new paradigm in healthcare.

The brain seems to be a tangle of wires

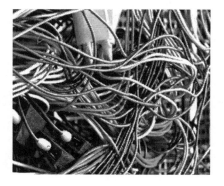

The brain makes it easy to target and change our wiring
Who would have thought that we could change our own wiring? Given that we each have about 100 billion neurons, each with up to 10,000 synapses, it would seem impossible to organize our wires. And it would be, except for the brain's amazing power to do it for us – automatically and rapidly.

Our wiring automatically organizes itself by stress level

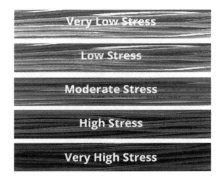

The brain has a built-in circuitry organizer, which makes that tangle of wires easier to control. It organizes our wires by stress level. When we're in a particular level of stress, all the wires that record our past responses at that stress level are available to us.

Based on evolutionary biology, we need to have instant access to wires (strings of neurons that form memories of past experiences) to replay quickly and easily. Instructions about how to get from each stress level to joy (or at least, a better state) are instantly accessible to us. When we access them, we stand a better chance of survival. For convenience, we have identified five levels of brain stress.

To make it easier to find a wire that is controlling us – and our eating and weight – we number these stress levels, or "brain states," ranging from very low stress to very high stress. If you are not very stressed right now, say low stress (Brain State 2), then the wires that tell you what to do when you are in Brain State 2 to meet your needs and reduce your stress are "hot" or "online." If there were a basket of bread on the table near you, it would activate memories of what you did in the past when you were in Brain State 2 and saw a basket of bread on the table. The wires from the other brain states would be "cold" or "offline" and they would not interfere with your decision about what to do.

We can number our stress levels for easy access to our wires

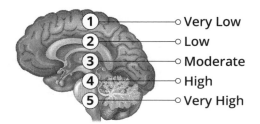

If you were highly stressed, in Brain State 5, and saw the bread, and had overeaten bread in the past when you were that stressed, it would activate your "stress eating" wire and you'd crave the bread and immediately start eating it! It is easier for you to replay old tapes with minimal energy – thereby speeding up response time, which is good for survival!

At each stress level, a different brain area is in charge

We are very different in each stress level because for each one, the brain assigns a different area to be in charge. If stress is very low, we need to think more rather than run from lions, so it assigns the top part of the brain to be in charge. As our stress increases, the area in charge becomes more primitive and, although it responds faster (fight or flight), it is usually more extreme, ineffective, and prone to overreaction.

The neocortex, which is our thinking brain and the seat of our consciousness, takes control when we are in low stress, whereas in high stress, the reptilian brain, the brain area given to extremes, is in charge. It's normal to spend time in all five stress levels in any day. There are no bad stress levels. However, becoming stuck in high stress causes most of our emotional, behavioral, and health problems.

At each number, a different brain area is in charge

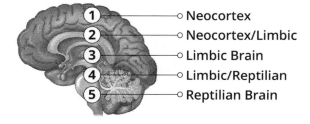

1. Neocortex
2. Neocortex/Limbic
3. Limbic Brain
4. Limbic/Reptilian
5. Reptilian Brain

We have a different basic need at each stress level

What is stress? It is the brain's wake-up call, telling us that we have an unmet need. This is the primary function of the brain: to alert us to meet our needs, so that we take action and not only survive but thrive.

At each level of stress, we have a different need. When we are in stress overload (Brain State 5), the brain is sure that we are going to die. We do not feel safe. The brain pulls out all the stops and unleashes a fight-or-flight drive to survive. Even if the stress is caused by a psychological hurt, such as someone rejecting us, the brain unleashes an overwhelming drive to find safety.

When we are at Brain State 4, we are definitely stressed. The brain looks for emotional connection, as our primary need is to emotionally connect to others for survival. Without that emotional connection, we would not have survived infancy. That connection was also necessary in order to survive during hunter-gatherer times. Our need in Brain State 4 is love.

What about Brain State 3? In Brain State 3 we are a little stressed. Perhaps we are anxious or thinking too much. We need to find some small ways to feel better. Our need in Brain State 3 is for comfort.

At each number, we have a different basic need

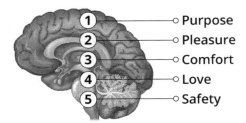

1 — Purpose
2 — Pleasure
3 — Comfort
4 — Love
5 — Safety

When we are at Brain State 2, we feel good, but not great. We are present and aware, but the brain's reward center is not activated. The brain demands that we not only ease our stress, but experience positive emotions and rewards. Our need in Brain State 2 is for pleasure.

And at Brain State 1, we feel great. We are present and aware and feel the glow of the activation of the brain's reward center. All five of our needs are met – and we can focus on our highest need: purpose.

Needs not met? The brain often encodes a stress eating wire

We have wires at each stress level that are enormously efficient in helping us meet our needs and return to joy. However, when a new situation arises and the brain can't find an effective wire, its easiest solution is to prompt us to overeat. By reaching for food at that time, we encode a stress eating wire.

Once encoded, the brain perceives the wire as effective and triggers it repeatedly. When we're stressed, we go right to food. Food does not meet our underlying need, but we use it anyway, as our wiring tells us to eat in that way. Although overeating is easy and a quick fix for stress, our underlying need continues to be unmet, which stresses us even more. The stressed brain continues to trigger overeating, and we may even eat more. This is the brain's way of asking, "How much do I have to eat in order to meet my need?"

The answer is that no amount of food will meet that need, because we are not eating for bodily needs. We are overeating to try to meet our emotional needs. Even if we ate all day and all night, overeating would not meet our primary emotional needs. When we are very stressed, we need safety. The brain is disconnected, so even if we are safe, we do not feel safe. When we are a little less stressed, we search for love. In less stressed states, our needs are for comfort, pleasure, or purpose. Overeating sugary, processed foods does not fulfill those needs, even though a wire tells us that it does!

Stuck in the Stress Eating Cycle

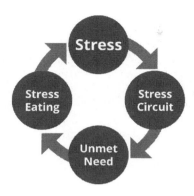

The problem is that we are now wired to stress eat and people tell us to stop overeating. That's ridiculous! We can't stop overeating when our wiring tells us to overeat. In fact, the more we force ourselves to go against our wiring and deny our unmet needs, the more stressed we become. Now we are stuck in a stress eating cycle. We're not sure why we are so hungry and so out of control. It's not us! It's that our wiring has caused us to be stuck in the stress eating cycle!

We can break the stress eating cycle!

Stopping overeating is so simple! The problem is that a wire is triggering us to overeat. It's blocking our natural drive to eat healthy. What do we do? We break that wire. Once that old rusty wire stops bothering us, we can honor our natural drive to eat healthy.

We can stop seeing our stress eating as a dietary problem. It's a wiring issue. We can focus on changing the wire that triggers us to overeat. It's a Stress Circuit (allostatic circuit), and we can begin to transform it into a Joy Circuit (homeostatic circuit) that helps us eat healthy and meet our needs.

Breaking Free from the Stress Eating Cycle

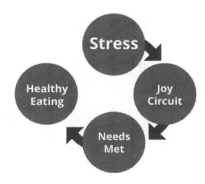

When we break that wire and step out of the stress eating cycle, legions of circuits that activate healthy eating begin taking charge. We start eating in a way that is in harmony with our evolutionary biology. Our ancestors were hungry when they ate. There were no processed foods back then, so they ate real, whole foods. What's more, our ancestors had no electricity or batteries, so they ate during the day and took a rest from food for about 12 hours. This food rest at night corresponds to what we know about how long it takes the body to burn up extra blood sugar (glucose) from the day's food intake, our body starch (glycogen), and begin to burn up body fat (triglycerides).

We have had that natural drive within us all the time. Now we have the tools to access it. We can rewire our brain wires so that we can eat that way intuitively, giving ourselves just the foods our body needs. Now we have a way to be at peace with food and with ourselves.

The 5 Eating Styles

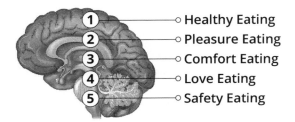

Identify your stress eating style, and rewire it!

The solution to overeating is to discover the wire that blocks you from your natural drive to eat healthy and break it. Then two seemingly miraculous things occur. You start eating healthy naturally and you feel free to meet your basic needs in ways that really work!

If your stress eating wire is pleasure eating, when the wire isn't bothering you anymore, you'll start feasting on natural pleasures. Your senses will come alive! Food will taste better, and what you hear, smell, touch, and see will deliver an abundance of pleasure.

If your style is to eat for comfort, once you've freed yourself of that wire, you'll find hundreds of ways to comfort yourself. Instead of using food for comfort, then having a food hangover or living in a carb fog, you'll notice that small acts of caring for yourself take hold. You enjoy being good to yourself in healthy ways. If your eating style is love, breaking that stress eating wire is so liberating! Now that food is no longer love, we become aware of the love inside us and tap into it, so that it's easier to give and receive love. Our relationships naturally deepen.

Last, if your stress eating style is safety, then breaking that wire transforms your life. The most common response to discovering this wire is a flooding of compassion for ourselves. Of course, we would have such strong drives to overeat. That wire told us food was the source of our safety, protection, existence, or security. We can exhale because we understand why the drive to overeat was so strong and why that wire made it impossible to stop stress eating.

The 5 Eating Solutions

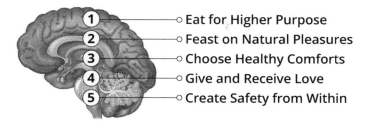

1. Eat for Higher Purpose
2. Feast on Natural Pleasures
3. Choose Healthy Comforts
4. Give and Receive Love
5. Create Safety from Within

By breaking that circuit, something deep inside us shifts. We connect to the deepest part of ourselves, our emotional and spiritual core. By doing so, we feel peace and power from within and nourish our spirits naturally and in ways that food never could.

It's a simple solution to stress eating
The plan is rather simple. You'll learn some emotional tools to short-circuit your stress eating and stop cravings, then move right into discovering your stress eating style and rewiring it. While you're at it, you will rewire three other circuits so that it's easier to eat healthy and release extra weight.

Before launching the plan, please reflect on the story of your eating and weight, assess your current level of joy, and personalize your practice of using the tools.

Tell Your Story

The prefrontal cortex loves to tell stories! A Stress Circuit often forms in a moment of stress overload. In a traumatic moment when the brain is overloaded, we escape from being present, encoding a circuit such as "I get my safety from binge-eating sweets." Also, other memories related to that situation encode circuits, often a "bundle" of them. These wires cause chronic stress, which ruins the prefrontal cortex's story about your life at that time or since.

The prefrontal cortex makes up a story and that story, no matter how negative or false it is, becomes part of our personal narrative. A major benefit of EBT is better understanding where we have been and really knowing ourselves, building self-compassion, and making good decisions about how we live our lives. We can understand the old story we told ourselves and encode a new, more reasonable one.

I had a life-changing event when my mother criticized my body and put me on a carb-free diet. My mind turns blank when I think of it. I retold the story and did about 10 Cycles. I have to process my emotions to see my mother clearly and forgive her.

I like to eat salty crunchy foods. When I rewired my Food Circuit, my brain brought up images of eating salty crunchy foods with my beloved Dad, who passed away when I was 12 years old. I got my love from compulsively eating foods I ate with him. I felt compassion for myself, and then rewired the circuit. It's time to stop living in the past.

**Tell the story of your
eating and weight.**

Please jot down some facts about your eating and weight history. Tell your story. Then, throughout the course, add to these notes. By the conclusion of this book, you can retell the story of your eating and weight in a way that eases your stress and helps you break free of the stress eating cycle.

Note from Kendra about eating and weight

I was so fat by age one that my mother was horrified. She was afraid that I would have "stovepipe" legs like my grandmother. I weighed 35 pounds by the age of one, and the weight alone may have encoded Stress Circuits.

My next notable weight gain was at about the age of 10 when my body started changing. I lost my innocence and my joy. I wanted to hide because I didn't know what to do about how boys were looking at me. I stuffed my feelings and started craving sugar. A Stress Circuit was probably encoded then, too.

During my first year of college, I was so anxious. My high school was small, and everyone knew each other, and then I enrolled in a sprawling university. I thought I had joy because I was drinking and binge eating dorm food, but I was so anxious. No wonder I gained about 20 pounds and never took it off. From then on, my weight was either stable or increasing.

Your notes about eating and weight

In this warm-up activity, please write about several times in your life when you started overeating or gained weight. Reflect on the changes, losses, or upsets that occurred within one year of that time. You'll fill in pieces of the puzzle as you move through this book, and by the conclusion, you'll have important insights into your story. For now, begin to tell the story of your eating and weight with as much or as little detail as feels comfortable to you. For information about downloading forms for this chapter and the rest of the book, see Your EBT Experience, page 277.

The Joy Inventory

To break free of overeating, we must become highly skilled at creating joy in our life regardless of circumstances. This is a skill and you can learn it.

That state of joy requires processing emotions (think of them as the "steam" that rises from stress) effectively, then moving forward in a purposeful way. That is fairly complicated! If we do good in the world and abuse or neglect ourselves, that's not sustainable! Accordingly, there are three sub-scales to this inventory. The first one assesses our effectiveness in meeting our fundamental needs. The next one checks the reasons for our actions based on the higher-order "eudonic" rewards. The last sub-scale measures how effective we are at emotional connection. If awareness of doing something for a higher-order reason is the silver medal of our spiritual evolution, then emotional connection is the gold.

During the next 30 days, please track your progress in meeting your needs and creating joy from purpose and connection, taking the Joy Inventory now and again at days 16 and 30 of the challenge.

 **Track your progress
in creating joy!**

The Joy Inventory

Needs

In the last week, how often did you meet each of your basic needs?

Purpose
    1 = Rarely   2 = Sometimes   3 = Often   4 = Very Often

Pleasure
    1 = Rarely   2 = Sometimes   3 = Often   4 = Very Often

Comfort
    1 = Rarely   2 = Sometimes   3 = Often   4 = Very Often

Love
    1 = Rarely   2 = Sometimes   3 = Often   4 = Very Often

Safety
    1 = Rarely   2 = Sometimes   3 = Often   4 = Very Often

Total Baseline Needs Score _____

Rewards

In the last week, how often did you experience these rewards?

Sanctuary: Peace and power from within
    1 = Rarely   2 = Sometimes   3 = Often   4 = Very Often

Authenticity: Feeling whole and being genuine
    1 = Rarely   2 = Sometimes   3 = Often   4 = Very Often

Vibrancy: Healthy with a zest for life
    1 = Rarely   2 = Sometimes   3 = Often   4 = Very Often

Integrity: Doing the right thing
    1 = Rarely   2 = Sometimes   3 = Often   4 = Very Often

Intimacy: Giving and receiving love
    1 = Rarely   2 = Sometimes   3 = Often   4 = Very Often

Spirituality: Aware of the grace, beauty, and mystery of life
    1 = Rarely   2 = Sometimes   3 = Often   4 = Very Often

Freedom: Common excesses fade
    1 = Rarely   2 = Sometimes   3 = Often   4 = Very Often

Total Baseline Rewards Score _____

Connection

In the last week, how often did you connect in this way?

Being aware that I can create joy
    1 = Rarely   2 = Sometimes   3 = Often   4 = Very Often

Choosing to create a moment of joy
    1 = Rarely   2 = Sometimes   3 = Often   4 = Very Often

Spiraling up from stress to joy
    1 = Rarely   2 = Sometimes   3 = Often   4 = Very Often

Enjoying sensory pleasures
    1 = Rarely   2 = Sometimes   3 = Often   4 = Very Often

Appreciating the joy of eating healthy food
    1 = Rarely   2 = Sometimes   3 = Often   4 = Very Often

Feeling the joy of releasing extra weight
    1 = Rarely   2 = Sometimes   3 = Often   4 = Very Often

Feeling love for myself
    1 = Rarely   2 = Sometimes   3 = Often   4 = Very Often

Feeling love for others
    1 = Rarely   2 = Sometimes   3 = Often   4 = Very Often

Feeling love for all living beings
    1 = Rarely   2 = Sometimes   3 = Often   4 = Very Often

Total Baseline Connection Score _____

The Joy Inventory Summary

Category	Baseline	Optimal Range
Needs	_____	15 to 20
Rewards	_____	21 to 28
Connection	_____	27 to 36
Total	_____	63 to 84

What is your amazing learning about your needs?

_____

What is your amazing learning about your rewards?

_____

What is your amazing learning about your connection?

_____

Setting Up Your EBT Practice

The purpose of this chapter is to help you set up a personal EBT practice. You are training your brain to process life in a highly effective way, which takes learning something new each day, practicing the tools, and for best results, using the tools with another person.

Learning: 10 Minutes Daily

Take 10 minutes per day to learn something new. The reptilian brain would be happy if you did not use the tools well, as it does not like change. However, by using the tools well, you become wired for joy more rapidly and see better results faster. Determine when you will do your 10 minutes of learning daily, and make it a habit. What if you want to take two days to do one day's activities or need a day off now and then? Take that time. This is your book and please personalize the pace to meet your needs.

I do my 10 minutes of learning when I wake up in the morning. My mind is fresh and I use the new ideas all day.

Check Ins: 10 Per Day

The Check In Tool interrupts the spontaneous firing of circuits that cause us stress and stops them from becoming stronger. In fact, each Check In weakens them and, at the same time, strengthens the circuits that spiral us up to joy. The Check In Tool is the master tool of EBT. As you progress in

Your EBT Daily Practice
- 10 minutes of learning
- 10 Check Ins
- 1 Connection

your training, you will use the Check In advanced skills that amplify your power to heal past hurts, rewire habits, and become wired for joy. The Check In Tool is the gateway to taking charge of your unconscious mind.

The EBT Practice includes checking in 10 times daily. Checking in takes 30 seconds to four minutes, depending on our stress level. These emotional tools are very quick in comparison to relaxation or cognitive tools, which take 20 or 30 minutes to accomplish the same relief.

When I check in a lot, my brain starts staying "checked in" automatically. Highly recommended!

Connections: One Per Day

You will experience better results faster if you use EBT with others by making connections, listening to others use the tools, and asking them to listen to you use the tools. The emotional brain is the social brain and allows the tools to go deeper into the brain when it is stabilized by another person listening to us.

Some people form their own EBT group through book clubs, neighborhood groups, or corporate study groups. Consider doing that.

Many others want more privacy, and an "instant" circle of support and join EBT telegroups at ebt.org. Telegroups are facilitated by Certified EBT Providers or Mentors and give you access to connections with five to seven other people. Our research has shown that these connections, along with weekly group sessions, or even more frequent sessions, spark more rewiring and better health outcomes than using this method on your own.

I have a 30-minute weekly telegroup with six people to connect with and my sister who lives in Connecticut to be another connection. She's doing the Joy Challenge, too. I have plenty of connections right now.

Connections are brief periods of practicing the tools between two people. In a telephone call that lasts one to five minutes, someone uses a tool or does a Check In. The reptilian brain calms down, and the tools become even more effective.

Connections are quick and effective. There is no chit-chat. While you may see these people as your friends, they are functioning as connection buddies, which can be even more important than friends. If you are a member of an EBT telegroup, your connection buddies have no idea who you are – no contact information is shared. All calls are made through our private EBT telephone system. No advice is given, and either party can conclude the connection at any time. Also, they have the same mission that you do – to conquer stress eating and raise their set point. Afterwards, both people go on with their day, radiating positive energy.

Now that you've set up your EBT Practice, let's look at the technology that can make it easy to integrate EBT into your daily life.

Using Tech to Connect

Although you can use this book without any technology, you will like EBT more and see better results if you use it. As a book owner, you receive a discount of 25% on our Online PLUS membership. Please see the coupon on page 278 for details. Questions? Email support@ebt.org.

EBT Technology
• The EBT App (iOS and Android)   • The EBT Website   • The EBT Phone System

The EBT App (iOS and Android)

The EBT App ("Connect by EBT") is designed to give you immediate access to the tools, anytime and anywhere. When we are stressed, the brain "forgets" to check in, and even if we have memorized the tool lead-ins, the brain cannot access those memories. The brain perceives the app as a separate entity, an outside source of support in tracking and using the tools. Develop a close relationship with the app, and your results from the Joy Challenge will be far better. It will soon become a habit to keep your EBT app with you and reach for it hourly, plus whenever you are stressed.

The EBT app includes relaxing audios, so you have stress relief in your pocket. If you join a telegroup, your app will give you one-touch access to your group members by telephone and messaging, and direct messaging with your Certified EBT Provider or Mentor.

The EBT Website

The EBT Website delivers all the features of the app, as well as many more. We recommend logging in daily to view the video demonstration that accompanies this book's content for each day. Also, take a minute or two to read a posting on the forum boards and leave a connecting message in response. Also, post your own comments, Cycles, and learnings.

The EBT Online Community is designed to give you a variety of ways to learn EBT. Check out the weekly live call-in workshops, listen to recordings of past sessions in which other participants do Cycles on just the challenge you are facing now. Want small group support and private community connections? Join a telegroup. If you have a particular circuit that is difficult to rewire or are dealing with a situation that is hard to resolve, schedule a 25-minute coaching session with the Certified EBT Provider of your choice. With their support, you can spiral up quickly!

The EBT Phone System

EBT has a private phone system. The emotional brain is extraordinarily sensitive to the sound of the human voice, so telephone communication is extremely powerful. You can use the EBT line for groups, coaching, workshops, and mentor sessions. The vocal experience is pure, as other people on the call cannot see you. Each person maintains privacy, yet verbal exchanges convey the range of tender, warm, and powerful human experience.

The EBT Phone System includes a special feature for using the tools when you do not have privacy. You just call in on your EBT phone line, select "1" and you will hear me guide you through a Check In. Select your brain state on your phone's keypad, and I will walk you through the appropriate tool. Spiral up to One rapidly and privately.

EBT Technology Support

Our EBT Support Team can help you set up and become comfortable with the technology. Our goal is to continuously improve our services and make EBT an even more life-changing experience for you. Please share your feelings and needs with us. We hope you enjoy this high-tech way to connect with yourself and others, and to raise your emotional set point.

Community Connections

- Two people meet by telephone for one to five minutes.
- Ask, "Is this a good time?"
- Plan the activity (use a tool, share an amazing learning or a Joy Point).
- One person speaks, using the lead-ins from the app, website, or book. The other listens.
- The person who listens gives a connecting message.
- The connection ends . . . Goodbye.
- If you have time left within the five minutes? Share another Joy Point and connecting message.

How do connections fit in?

You connect with people who you intend to know over time. If they are members of your telegroup, you can get to know them slowly, being with them in the weekly or daily group, and connecting with them as you feel comfortable doing so. The weekly or daily telegroup session serves as an anchor for the group, with structure, inspiration, and shared experiences.

All connections are by voice, as the brain craves the sound of the human voice, and the sound of the voice activates legions of feel-good emotional wires. Oddly enough, when you listen to a voicemail from a connection buddy, your brain processes it as if that person were connecting with you in real time. Although the EBT electronic message system can be very convenient, we also make it very easy to make voice connections for one reason: the brain changes far more rapidly when we make them!

Innovative Ways to Connect

- Call and leave a Joy Point.
- Record a quick Cycle on their voicemail.
- Say 10 Grind Ins on their voicemail.
- Share your amazing learning on their voicemail.
- Do the Damage Control Tool on their voicemail.
- Call your buddy back and leave a connecting message.
- Call and speak with them in real time for Grind Ins.
- Read a written Cycle to them.
- Use the Flow Tool (3 Tool) with them.
- Do coursework together ("Kit Buddies") – call to coordinate, hang up, you both take 10 minutes to work, then call back to share your amazing learnings.
- Practice A+ Anger, so your Cycles go deeper.
- Do Cycles and give connecting messages.
- Call during a work break and say, "I have three minutes. What do you want to do?"
- Guide each other through a Check In.

What is a connecting message?

Have you noticed that right after you open up to someone, you feel a bit stressed? We noticed that, too, and to move through that stress, we invented connecting messages.

The person that listens to you use the tools is a warm presence and does not give advice. They give you the ultimate gift of listening to you without judgment, then saying a few kind words to you that they think will be nurturing for you to hear and they feel safe saying. You use lead-ins from the app, website, or book to guide your way in making these exchanges brief, safe, and rewarding.

Examples of Community Connections

Ring. Ring.

Denny: Hi Carla. Is this a good time?

Carla: *Yes, I have about two minutes.*

Denny: Great. That's perfect.

Carla: *What about sharing a Joy Point or doing a Check In together?*

Denny: Sure, I'd like to listen to you share a Joy Point, if you're up for it.

Carla: *Okay. I had a big Joy Point today when my dog had puppies – four of them!*

Denny: When you did your work, the feeling and sensations in my body were . . . a big smile. The way your work was a gift to me was . . . I have been stalled on my project, and now I feel like doing it.

Carla: *Bye. "See" you in group tomorrow.*

Denny: Great. See you then. Bye.

Ring. Ring.

Theresa: Hi Miguel. Is this a good time?

Miguel: *Yes, I'm glad you called. I can't find my Mood Circuit.*

Theresa: Do you want to work on it?

Miguel: *Yes, I want to do a quick Cycle.*

Theresa: Great.

Miguel: *The situation is that I am always in a bad mood. I fly off the handle and don't think about what I'm saying. I know I scare people and my wife hates it when I'm that way. What I'm most stressed about is . . . I fly off the handle. I feel angry that I fly off the handle. I can't stand it that I fly off the handle. I HATE it that I fly off the handle. I HATE IT!!! . . . My mind just went blank. I must have unlocked the circuit. I feel sad that . . . I lose it sometimes. I feel afraid that I am hurting my marriage. I feel guilty that I keep on flying off the handle. I feel guilty that I go on acting hostile. Of course I do that, because my unreasonable expectation is . . . I get my . . . safety from . . . being hostile. Hmmmmm. That rings true. That feels right. I discovered my Mood Circuit!*

Theresa: When you did your work, the feeling and sensations in my body were . . . fear and guilt, because I fly off the handle too, but also, security, that I am not alone. The way your work was a gift to me was . . . I realized that I judge myself for flying off the handle. I am going to stop judging myself. Thank you for helping me see that.

Miguel: *Thanks.*

Theresa: I feel better. Thanks for the connection.

Miguel: *Bye.*

Theresa: Bye.

Connecting Messages

- Be supportive but do not analyze, praise, or in any way be "parental." Instead, be open and intimate, just what the emotional brain needs most!

- Share the feelings and sensations you had while listening. The other person has been vulnerable. You are vulnerable back – it's a two-way street.

- This is a highly effective message: "The way your work was a gift to me was that your expressing anger inspired me to try. Expressing anger has been hard for me. Thank you!" This is less effective: "The way your work was a gift to me was that I learned a lot."

- Use these lead-ins to guide your way:

  When you did your work, the feelings and sensations in my body were . . . (e.g., I felt worried, then I smiled and felt happy.)

  The way your work was a gift to me was . . . (e.g., that I learned a lot about how to express joy because that is hard for me.)

Community Guidelines

Safety is our first priority. It is the responsibility of each member to take care of their own safety, and to create safety right away if for any reason an EBT experience does not feel comfortable. The community guidelines help create a safe, warm environment.

The EBT Community Guidelines

- Make no judgments.
- Offer no unasked-for advice.
- Do not interrupt.
- Be a warm presence for others.
- Do not mention other programs or products.
- Support privacy and confidentiality.

Great work – and on to the next step

You have completed the introduction to The Joy Challenge. You are now prepared to have a wonderful time learning the EBT method. Start with Day 1: Begin with Joy in Mind. Enjoy seeing how rapidly you can change and savor your unique journey through the Joy Challenge!

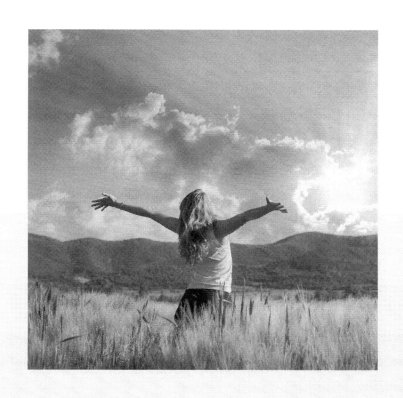

Spiral Up
to Joy

Day 1. Begin with Joy in Mind

Joy is the state in which our brain is in harmony and we are chemically at our best. Our basic needs: safety, love, comfort, pleasure, and purpose, are fully met. In that state, we eat healthy naturally and release weight. Joy can be created. It's a brain skill, and we will strengthen that skill today.

Happiness is not the same as joy. All joyful states are happy, but not all happy states are joy. You can be happy because you eat ice cream, spend money, or down a few drinks. These are artificial pleasures which tend to "wear out" the brain's reward center. They are not bad or wrong, but they do not bring us joy. The brain insists on joy and any of these joy substitutes eventually adds to our stress rather than bringing us to our joy.

The Many Signs of Joy

Joyful	In Awe	Aware	Grateful	Anchored
Glowing	Hopeful	Open	Secure	Connected
Warmed	Loving	Present	Amused	Comforted
Peaceful	Forgiving	Happy	Safe	Compassionate
Playful	Energized	Inspired	Creative	Expansive

Joy is designed to give us a natural high that is still grounded in reality, rather than a false high or numbness that is followed by an unnecessary low. All joy includes a trace of pain, which adds to the magnitude of the pleasure. Much like adding a squeeze of lemon to sugar water, natural pleasures include an awareness that this moment will not last.

Joy is more than mere happiness, which can become addictive and rather flat. It is the ultimate chemical elixir. You know you are in joy when you smile broadly, feel a wave of relaxation run through your body, and sense the deeper meanings of life.

When I see my puppy, I feel so much love, but also a slight awareness that she will not always be with us. That makes me cherish the moment even more.

I watch the blazing sunset and am enchanted, but part of me knows that the colors will fade. That reality grounds me in the preciousness of life and brings me intense joy, even with the slight grieving I do.

This "joy" experience is rooted in delivering us intense natural pleasure only when it is good for us, and good for the survival of the species. The multi-layered emotions and sensations arrive by using the brain's optimal pathways, which we mirror by using the EBT tools. Joy is available to all of us, but it is not for sale. It is free to us when we use the tools, and when we do, stress eating ceases. We have no need to overeat because our needs are so fully met by that natural state.

The reptile is not happy about joy
This entire discussion of joy may make you stressed. Joy feels fabulous, but it is a threat to the reptilian brain. The more your brain is in the stress habit with a set point in stress, the more it will resist joy and cause backlashes.

As you move up your brain's set point, you'll become comfortable with times when the reptilian brain triggers stress for a health-promoting reason. You are moving away from chronic stress. The reptile is not happy. It likes everything to stay the same, including your set point. Keep your sense of humor. The war has just begun, and with your passion and persistence, you will win! After all, it's just a reptile!

I started seeing joy everywhere, even while sitting in a stale meeting. I was surprised at the pleasure I had from rubbing my neck or thinking about how much I love my boyfriend. I started creating so much joy that my lizard brain had a backlash. Nothing looked good to me, then it passed. I understand that this is a war!

Why
The more moments we spend in joy, the more we train the brain for joy. The emotional brain ONLY learns by experiences; knowledge, insight, planning, and deciding do not reach the emotional brain.

Just like children do what their parents do, not what they say, the emotional brain is the messy, oppositional, confused, and rebellious child within. When we feed it experiences of spiraling up to joy, all those shenanigans stop and we have peace from within. The brain releases the stress habit and adopts the joy habit.

How
Begin your day by stating, "I am creating JOY in my life." This declaration activates every major circuit in the brain. It's a revolutionary statement, implying: I matter. I have the power to create. Joy is not just for other people, but for me, and my life is important.

As you move through your day, watch for moments of joy. Create moments of joy, when your body relaxes into a slight glow of positive emotions. There are three evidence-based ways to create these surges of neurotransmitters:

Bring up a happy memory

Bring to mind any happy memory, often it's a loving moment, a happy reunion, or an experience of intense natural pleasure. Notice that you feel a wave of relaxation and a glow. Remind yourself, "Joy Point."

Enjoy a sensory pleasure

Any natural pleasure that our hunter-gatherer ancestors used to reward themselves can instantly activate a relaxation response and a joy response. Whether it is watching a sunset, slipping into a warm bath, stroking your own body, or hugging a loved one, it can bring a sense of well-being. Score a Joy Point!

Engage in a kind act

Do something nice. Even if it is just smiling at someone, sending a warm email, or checking with a loved one about how they feel and what they need, you'll experience a warm glow – a Joy Point.

My best friend tracks calories, grams, and steps to lose weight. I count Joy Points!

Create a Joy Point
• Bring up a happy memory.
• Enjoy a sensory pleasure.
• Engage in a kind act.

Score three Joy Points before sleeping

Before you go to sleep, say again the purpose of your day: "I am creating joy in my life." If you like, bring three Joy Points that you created today to mind – this delivers three more Joy Points.

The Success Check

This book is based on mastering one small but important skill each day for 30 days. This requires practicing each skill in a focused, intensive way. By using a skill repeatedly for one day, your brain will change and be ready to learn the next day's skill.

The daily Success Check helps you track your progress. Check off what you have accomplished that day. Take an extra day if you need it. Do not go on to the next activity until you have checked off all the items on the Success Check.

By the conclusion of this course, you will amaze yourself at how rapidly you have reset your brain and your relationship with food. Record your biggest accomplishment in EBT each day, what you are most proud of having done. Also, record your biggest challenge in EBT, what you want to focus on the next day to experience the best results. You will probably learn something each day that fascinates you. That is your amazing learning. Record one daily.

Morning Check In:
- State, "I am creating joy in my life."

Throughout the Day:
- Create 10 Joy Points.

Evening Check In:
- State, "I am creating joy in my life."
- Bring to mind three moments of joy from your day.

You can create joy in your life. It's a skill. Think of it as your "joy muscle" and work it! You don't have to do this perfectly to see remarkable results. Have fun doing it, and celebrate each small but important step you take in amplifying your joy!

Success Check Day 1

- **Daily Success**

☐ In the morning, I declared, "I am creating joy in my life."

☐ I created 10 Joy Points.

☐ In the evening, I celebrated, saying, "I am creating joy in my life," and brought to mind three moments of joy from my day.

☐ I made one or more community connections to share Joy Points.

- **Did I pass the Success Check?   YES   NO**

If you did not, stay with this activity for one more day, then move on.

- **My Amazing Learning:**

_____

- **My Biggest Accomplishment:**

_____

- **My Biggest Challenge:**

_____

Congratulations!

**You have completed Day 1 of The Joy Challenge.
Your next step is Day 2. The 30-Second Check In.**

Day 2. The 30-Second Check In

You are becoming skilled at creating joy, however you might notice a hunger for a deeper connection to yourself. It is our present-moment connection to the deepest part of ourselves that we crave.

The Check In Tool, which we will start using today, will help you cut through the emotional stress of the moment, and connect with yourself. It is a practical tool that gives you access to rewiring your unconscious mind, but it is a sacred tool, too. When you use your thinking brain (prefrontal cortex) to check in with the deepest part of yourself, profound changes occur.

The 30-Second Check In
• **Connect your neocortex and emotional brain.** • **Automatically tap into your inner strength and wisdom.** • **Choose to experience joy and the goodness of life.**

I felt so connected to myself yesterday. Then, last night I had no desire to overeat. Fascinating!

Today, continue with your Joy Practice. Start your day by declaring, "I am creating joy in my life!" During the day, collect 10 Joy Points. Add to your practice the Check In Tool that gives you access to taking charge of your unconscious mind and rewiring your relationship with yourself.

Why

The deepest joys are all based on what we achieve internally, not our circumstances. However, the emotional brain only allows us to connect within as deeply as it is safe to connect. The more often we connect within emotionally, really experiencing our body and ourself, the deeper it will allow us to go. With each circuit we clear, we go deeper, which is why EBT is a progressive practice and why your EBT practice will become more rewarding over time.

Emotional connection is the pathway

Starting today, you will be accessing your emotions in a more robust and powerful way. Most of us process life by thinking. That's changing! Now we access our emotions 10 or more times per day.

By surrendering our thoughts to the more vivid world of emotions, we relinquish control over which feelings we feel. That's not a problem. Sure, negative ones arise first as the brain's way of alerting us to a real or perceived threat. Only by feeling our negative emotions does the brain relax and deliver to us the authentic, robust, and gritty positive emotions. It rewards us for turning on the spigot of negative emotions with a burst of positive ones.

In the grand benevolence of the emotional brain, negative emotions are our pathway to emotional growth. Each time we stay present to our emotions, we automatically update our unreasonable expectations that guide our drives, behaviors, and rewards. Effectiveness in feeling our negative emotions is the solution!

The elevated emotions make us unstoppable

The multi-layered elevated emotions – love, compassion, gratitude, hope, forgiveness, awe, and joy – make us exceedingly strong, able to fulfill our unique mission in life. These emotions are not like the false highs from artificial rewards (alcohol, sugar, drugs, and the thousands of "go-tos" enshrined in our Stress Circuits). They are grounded in reality, which enables our prefrontal cortex to open up to new ideas, challenges, and possibilities that we could not fathom only moments before.

This is the adventure of EBT! All you need do is stay the course. Do not quit. Appreciate that you are learning how to work with your emotional brain. It will take time, but each use of the tools – no matter how seemingly successful or unsuccessful it is – makes a productive mark on your unconscious mind. You will feel the difference and so will those around you.

When I check in, I feel a slight fear. I am accustomed to overthinking everything and I am not sure I want to connect with my emotions. I don't know what I'll find there, but I don't like the idea of being checked out. I will give it a try.

I can feel my emotions already and feel pretty connected to myself. I am eager to find ways that are more efficient in connecting and taking me to some more profound emotions. I am IN!

How

Just follow the simple steps below. If you are using the EBT app, it will guide you through three evidence-based techniques to rapidly reduce stress and will record your stats based on your combined Check Ins from both the app and website. Begin by clicking on the Check In icon on your app or following the instructions below:

Step 1: Take a deep breath

Begin by turning your attention to your body and your breathing. Take a deep breath and focus on breathing in so that your stomach rises up, and then exhale – a long, complete outbreath. This is **diaphragmatic breathing**. It's unnatural, and unnatural activities require that we turn our attention away from the buzzing thoughts in our thinking brain. The long exhale eases stress and activates the brain's reward center.

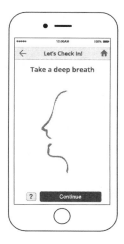

Step 2: Gently assume "Body at 1"

Next, change your posture and facial expression to the universal power positions. This gives your brain the message that you are in a state of well-being. Sit up or stand up tall, then put your shoulders back and your chest out. Next, lift up your chin a little, then stretch the corners of your mouth back toward your ears in a slight smile, and either warm your eyes with a loving expression or crinkle them as if you are laughing. Sustaining this for two minutes reduces the stress hormone cortisol by 25 percent and raises testosterone. It is called **proprioceptive posturing**.

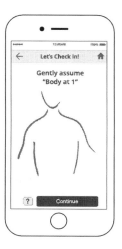

Step 3: Warmly observe yourself

Last, imagine throwing one cell of your being high up in the air and warmly observing yourself in the present moment, just as you are and without judgment. See yourself in this situation and notice a connection. You are connecting with yourself. This is important. Your thinking brain, the overseer of your emotional brain, is seeing you, hearing you, and feeling your feelings. That amounts to what we all need: a secure connection within.

This connection is your relationship with yourself. You might notice yourself using a nurturing inner voice. You may feel compassion for yourself. Your unconditional love for yourself – even a slight amount of it – makes a huge difference in your brain functioning and every aspect of your life in that moment. When you complete Step 3, notice that your body is more relaxed, and you are aware of a slight glow. You have checked in!

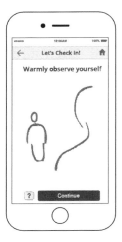

Choose your Check In plan

There are two plans for checking in. One plan is the basic plan, checking in hourly, that is, 10 times per day. Set your alarm or notification hourly to remind yourself to check in. The advantage of this plan is that you only have to check in 10 times.

The other plan is the easy plan, checking in every 30 minutes. The advantage of the easy plan is that you stay connected all day. Rather than giving stress time to activate a Stress Circuit, sustain stress overload, and block your joy, you prevent that circuit from taking hold.

I liked the every-30-minute Check In better right away. It was so much easier to stay checked in and have that glow in my body much of the day.

This easy, frequent Check In keeps the Stress Triangle in the brain from switching into "weight gain" and "constantly hungry" modes. Another advantage of checking in every 30 minutes is that the frequency helps the brain learn to check in automatically. With enough practice (much like going to the emotional gym), the brain begins to stay "checked in" spontaneously more of the time.

Encoding a strong, nurturing inner voice

Starting tomorrow, we will use lead-ins to amplify the power of this 30-Second Check In. In preparation for that next step, please begin thinking about your relationship with yourself. That internal dialog – the connection between your conscious mind and your unconscious mind – is the most significant predictor of the quality of your life. We use the EBT Tools to radically improve the effectiveness of that fundamental connection.

30-Second Check In

- **Take a deep breath.**
  Turn your attention to your belly and your breathing, pushing out your stomach as you inhale, followed by a long release.

- **Gently assume "Body at 1."**
  Shoulders back, chest out, chin up a little, a slight smile, and the expression of happiness or love in your eyes.

- **Warmly observe yourself.**
  Observe yourself, liking the person you see, and feeling a wave of compassion for yourself.

For now, consider giving your emotional brain a name. Common examples are the reptile within, the lizard brain, my rebellious brain, the little kid within me, and my "hell-on-wheels" brain. Also, common are more spiritual names, such as the deepest part of me, my inherent strength, goodness, and wisdom, my essence, my spirit, my soul, the God within me, or even the sanctuary in my body. Also, what voice will you use to speak to that brain? It's a relationship, so you might need different voices at different times, depending upon the needs of your emotional brain. You might want to use a tender, loving inner voice, a cheerleader voice, a prayerful voice, a strong voice, or a good parent voice. Give your emotional brain just the vocal tone and the words it needs to hear in that moment!

I used a loving voice after a binge, and I heard myself say to myself, "That's okay, Sweetie. It's not you. It's just a wire. You can rewire it when you are ready to do that." I felt the glow of joy in my body. It worked!

My lizard brain is so rebellious today, so I kindly but clearly told it to stop judging so much, to minimize the harm. I reassured it that life is difficult but these hard times will pass. My stress dissolved.

Enjoy the 30-Second Check In and notice that you feel present and connected to your body – just what evolutionary biology designed.

Success Check Day 2

- **Daily Success**

☐ I continued my Joy Practice, declaring, "I am creating joy in my life," morning and evening and scoring 10 Joy Points.

☐ I used the 30-Second Check In every 30 or 60 minutes.

☐ I made one or more community connections for support with the 30-Second Check In.

- **Did I pass the Success Check?   YES   NO**

If you did not, stay with this activity for one more day, then move on.

- **My Amazing Learning:**

_____

- **My Biggest Accomplishment:**

_____

- **My Biggest Challenge:**

_____

Congratulations!

**You have completed Day 2 of The Joy Challenge.
Your next step is Day 3. What's My Number?**

Day 3. What's My Number?

The 30-Second Check In is highly effective. Now let's build on that skill for times when stress is higher or you want more control over your brain state. To use the precise pathway to feel better faster takes identifying your stress level or brain state.

After using the 30-Second Check In yesterday, you may have noticed that your emotional brain's stress level varies a lot. This is normal.

You can identify your stress level and, like lock and key, use a tool that moves you through your brain's "optimal resiliency pathway" for that state, so you feel better faster!

> ## My brain state varies a lot.
> ## What's my number?

The reason our brain state changes a lot is that the brain is trying to detect how threatened we are. It wants our needs for safety, love, comfort, pleasure, and purpose to be met. If they are not, then it registers that we're in danger and it shifts gears to be sure that we have access to just the past experiences (wires) that will tell us what we did before when we were in that level of stress. It changes our brain state.

All this happens without our conscious awareness, which is one of the beauties of our evolutionary biology. The level of threat it perceives may be very different than the actual threat level we face, as it shifts gears based on psychological stress, which accounts for most of our stress.

What else impacts our brain state? Any physical pain impacts it, and so does metabolic stress, the blood sugar lows that follow the extreme highs brought about by eating processed, sugary foods. With psychological, physical, and metabolic stress all impacting our brain state, it's normal for it to change rapidly and for us to be in all five brain states in any given day.

Why

Checking your brain state to figure out your "stress number" will give you far more precision in understanding yourself, and spiraling up to joy.

I felt pretty good, or so I thought. Then I checked in and realized that I was at Brain State 3, almost Brain State 4. I used the tool for Brain State 3 and spiraled up to joy. My desire to eat sweets vanished!

Why is identifying the state of the brain – our stress level – so helpful?

1. We experience ourselves differently in all five levels
Celebrate that you are five different people – and so is everyone else! Our moods, behaviors, thinking, perceptions, and sensations vary widely depending on our brain state. Our brain state impacts our entire physiology and every aspect of life!

2. We activate different wires or memories in each state
In each brain state, our memories from past experiences in that state are "hot" or "online." Most of our responses are replays of the past. Each replay impacts how we feel, what we expect, and what we do. The brain convinces us these feelings, expectations, and responses are reasonable, even if they are not!

3. Each brain state has a different resiliency pathway
To return to joy, we must process our emotions effectively. We have five highly effective but very different resiliency pathways. To stop stress eating, we just use our resiliency pathways. We identify our brain state and use the tool for that state!

The brain stores circuits in five drawers, one for each stress level

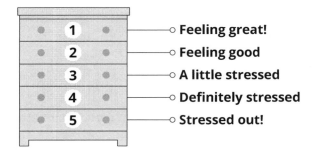

1 —○ **Feeling great!**
2 —○ **Feeling good**
3 —○ **A little stressed**
4 —○ **Definitely stressed**
5 —○ **Stressed out!**

4. If you know your brain state, you can understand yourself better

By being aware of our brain state, we can better understand ourselves and keep our sense of humor. We are so different in each brain state! Our brain state explains a lot about why we feel, think, and act the way we do. We can have more compassion for ourselves and stop self-judgment by knowing our brain state. The problem is not us, but our brain state, which has been triggered by our wires.

Brain States Impact Every Aspect of Life

State	Thoughts	Feelings	Relationships	Behavior
1	Abstract	Joyous	Intimate	Optimal
2	Concrete	Balanced	Companionable	Healthy
3	Rigid	Mixed	Social	Moderate
4	Reactive	Unbalanced	Needy/Distancing	Unhealthy
5	Irrational	Overwhelmed	Merged/Disengaged	Destructive

The preceding table shows four very diverse areas of life: thoughts, feelings, relationships, and behavior. Brain state impacts all of these areas. When we are in Brain State 1, these areas are functioning well. We are activating the circuits in the top drawer of the brain in which the neocortex is in charge. In addition, when we are at Brain State 1, we are remarkably like other people at Brain State 1: happy, healthy, connected, and intuitive.

When I'm at Brain State 1, I'm patient, kind, creative, and productive. At Brain State 5? I'm none of those things. Imagine that we are all like this. It's universal!

With each brain state below the optimal functioning of Brain State 1, performance in these areas deteriorates. We are activating circuits encoded from past experiences of stress and "replaying" them. Our more primitive brain areas take charge. In addition, the more stressed we are, the more our specific characteristics differ. In the 5th Drawer of the brain, in which the reptilian brain is in charge, we are all extreme and function poorly. One person might be hostile in that state, and another person might be numb. Even though the characteristics differ, they are equally extreme and ineffective.

Our brain states change without our awareness or approval. This means that for no clear reason, we can feel satisfied one minute, and have no desire to overeat. However, in the very next moment, for no logical reason, the brain can shift gears from Brain State 1 to Brain State 5. In that state, we may have a scarcity panic – we believe we have to have junk food or we will die! It is not logical, but it is how the brain works!

The Check In Tool

- Take a deep breath.
- Assume "Body at 1."
- Warmly observe yourself.
- What's my number?
  - 1 = Feeling Great!
  - 2 = Feeling Good
  - 3 = A Little Stressed
  - 4 = Definitely Stressed
  - 5 = Stressed Out!

5. Brain states control our eating styles

Understanding our brain state is tremendously helpful in stopping overeating. The drive to eat is extremely sensitive to stress. Once we know we are in a stressed brain state, and feel as if we are going to die if we don't overeat, we appreciate that the drive is a result of stress. We understand ourselves better.

It's essential to keep our sense of humor about our rather mixed-up brain, because the more stress we are in, the less likely we are to manage our eating well. At Brain State 5, we have very low impulse control. Our internal "good parent" (neocortical brain) goes on vacation. It disconnects from the "kids" (emotional brain). It loses control of reading our hunger signals accurately and shutting off the Stress Circuits that are telling us to overeat.

We've been using the 30-Second Check In to reconnect the thinking and emotional brains so we are present and in charge of our eating and ourselves. That process of connecting to ourselves and then staying connected is what keeps our stress eating styles (those wires) from being activated. If they are not activated, our Stress Triangle does not start spewing chemicals that cause hunger, cravings, lethargy, and weight gain. Staying present and emotionally connected is so important to stopping overeating and activating both healthy eating and natural weight loss that we are adding a new technique today to make it easier to do. We are identifying our brain state.

How

To use the Check In Tool, just add one step to your 30-Second Check In. Ask yourself, "What's my number?" There is an important part to doing this – you guess.

Why is guessing so important? Guessing is fun. Fun reduces our stress and with less stress, our thinking brain can stay connected to our emotional brain, which is the brain that brings out our inherent strength, goodness, and wisdom! We are really smart, really intuitive creatures, as long as we stay out of stress and don't think too much!

Effective Check Ins

- Guess your brain state. *Do not overthink it!*
- No judgments. Each brain state has advantages.
- Be curious. Your state can change quickly!

I guessed that I was at Brain State 5 when I was craving sweets after dinner. That helped me. The reptile was in charge and that lizard brain loves artificial rewards. That makes perfect sense.

I love my wife, but sometimes when she won't stop talking, I feel like a caged animal. I want to get away and de-stress. I checked in and realized that I was at Brain State 4. Of course I was distancing. That's stress for you.

When you check in, do not think about your stress level. Instead, ask yourself, "What's my number?" A number will come to mind, in essence, a "guess." Trust this initial answer to that question. Then, after you guess your brain state, score a Joy Point. Feel a surge of relaxation and pleasure in your body for one reason: you chose a number! At that moment, *the activity for today is complete.*

You do not need to change your brain state actively. You just need to play around with guessing your brain state and no matter what it is, not judging it. Judgments cause stress and stress causes overeating! Enjoy this special day of guessing your brain state.

Success Check Day 3

- **Daily Success**

☐ I continued my Joy Practice.

☐ I checked in 10 or more times and guessed my brain state.

☐ I made one or more community connections for support with guessing my brain state.

- **Did I pass the Success Check?   YES   NO**

If you did not, stay with this activity for one more day, then move on.

- **My Amazing Learning:**

_____

- **My Biggest Accomplishment:**

_____

- **My Biggest Challenge:**

_____

Great Progress!

**You have completed Day 3 of The Joy Challenge.
Your next step is Day 4. Let Feelings Flow.**

Day 4. Let Feelings Flow

Starting today, you'll be learning how to spiral up through stress to joy quickly.

I used the Flow Tool and stopped ruminating about the argument I had with my husband last night. I called him and told him that I loved him. I love this tool.

The tool we will learn today is the 3 Tool. It's so easy, powerful, and fascinating to use that most people use it throughout the day. The 3 Tool turns negative emotions into positive ones in about two minutes. It activates our reward center and shuts off stress.

The reason this tool works so well is that if you are a little stressed (Brain State 3), you are at the "tipping point." You are not activating an allostatic (stress) circuit that keeps you stuck in some form of stress, nor are you activating a homeostatic (joy) circuit.

You have a lot of power in that state. If you take that power and move through your slightly negative emotions, your brain will reward you with some gently positive ones. What's more, you'll be in a high brain state, running Joy Circuits and out of the territory that triggers stress eating.

Why

Use this tool for four reasons: 1) shut off stress eating on the spot; 2) turn negative emotions into positive ones; 3) avoid triggering a Stress Circuit which would put the reptile in charge; and 4) train your brain to be highly emotionally fluid. Emotional fluidity is a sought-after characteristic. By repeatedly using our natural resilience pathways, the brain gets in the habit of moving through negative emotions effectively (not suppressing them) and accessing robust, gritty, grounded joy.

Instead of planning what I eat and trying to control my appetite, I control my brain state. I spiral up from Brain State 3 to Brain State 1, and I feel completely satisfied on about a third less food. Interesting!

The Tipping Point

Comfort eating?

Use The 3 Tool to spiral up to One.

Switch your eating style naturally.

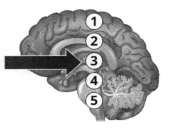

How

This is an easy tool. If you use it with excellent technique, it can almost always land you in Brain State 1. The entire world looks different from there, and the Stress Triangle ("Weight Central") in your brain activates healthy chemicals that shut off the desire to overeat, and create vibrancy – you feel healthy with a zest for life!

Pause between lead-ins

To use the 3 Tool, following the app, website, or book, state the first lead-in, or phrase. Then pause and wait for words to appear in your mind to complete the sentence. Pause again. Feel that feeling until it fades. Feeling the feeling is what heals us and brightens our mood.

The 3 Tool – Flow Tool	
• I feel angry that . . .	• I feel grateful that . . .
• I feel sad that . . .	• I feel happy that . . .
• I feel afraid that . . .	• I feel secure that . . .
• I feel guilty that . . .	• I feel proud that . . .

Next, state another lead-in . . . pause . . . and once again, feel the feeling until it fades. Continue this process for all eight feelings. **The pause makes all the difference**, as it prompts the thinking brain to connect with the emotional brain. That emotional connection between the two brains is the source of our safety and power. Imagine that! Our safety comes from a brain connection that we can achieve in real-time throughout the day!

Check the impact on your appetite

This tool takes about two minutes. You'll be more motivated to use it if you check your hunger level before and after using it. It is a great appetite suppressant! Try it before, during, and after eating.

My mind wandered to food and I started analyzing whether I should let myself eat lunch even though it was mid-morning. I checked in and realized that I was a little stressed, so I used the 3 Tool. I wasn't hungry anymore. What I had really needed was to de-stress.

Evenings are a challenge. I stay connected to myself all day because I'm vigilant. I want to stay at Brain State 1 to do right by my customers. In the evening, I forget about checking in and am stressed enough to eat chips late at night. I'm going to use this tool hourly, because it's easy to use and returns me to joy.

What if no words appear in your mind?

What if no words bubble up to complete the sentence? Just go on to the next lead-in. What if a couple lead-ins do not prompt your brain to express a feeling? Chances are you are not in Brain State 3. We'll learn tools for the other states starting tomorrow.

How do I know if I am too stressed to use this tool?

The words that appear in your mind for the first four lead-ins will all be on the same subject. That's a sign that you are at Brain State 4 and may need the 4 Tool (the "Cycle Tool"). We'll learn it soon.

How do I know if I am not stressed enough to use this tool?

If you feel present and aware but no words appear in your mind when you state the first four lead-ins, you could be in any of the states! Sometimes the brain does that. However, it's quite common that when we are in Brain State 2, feelings do not flow. You can state one feeling, but a flow of feelings? Most strong emotions come from stress. They are the "steam" that comes off a circuit. You may not be stressed enough to use this tool. You may be better off with the Brain State 2 Tool. We'll learn that tool soon.

The order of the feelings in the 3 Tool matters

The order of the feelings mirrors the brain's natural emotional processing. Use the lead-ins exactly as shown. For best results, do not change the order.

Enjoy knowing the contents of your unconscious mind

The words that appear in your mind come from pouring out the contents of circuits that were encoded long ago. They do not have to make sense. Do not analyze your feelings. Feel them. Enjoy this fascinating, deeper knowledge of yourself.

I used the Flow Tool and said, "I feel angry that . . ." and the words that appeared in my mind were: my sister is so critical of me. I had no idea I was stressed about that. I felt compassion for myself and for my sister. We grew up in a household where being critical of each other was considered a loving act. We were "helping" each other with self-improvement. I like this tool!

Oh my gosh, I'm at Brain State 1!

As you move through each of the eight lead-ins, notice the changing sensations in your body. If you started at Brain State 3, more often than not you will find yourself at Brain State 1.

Do you have a missing feeling?

Most of us have one of the eight core emotions that is challenging to express. That's your missing feeling. Make it easier to feel that feeling by adding the words "a little" to the lead-in. For example, "I feel *a little* secure that . . ." Adding them to the tool will train your brain that it's safe to feel that missing feeling, and soon you will be quite effective at expressing it.

My missing feeling is happiness. I know how to reward myself with carbs, but feeling happy? I'm not sure exactly what that means. I hope my brain will become more comfortable with me feeling real happiness, not stretching myself to feel happy when I know I am not.

The special power of guilt

Guilt is the most common missing feeling. Perhaps we were raised in a stressed environment in which we had to be perfect to feel loved. Expressing guilt in that environment would not be safe. Guilt is not shame. Shame is "I am a bad person." Guilt is "My behavior could use some improvement . . ." Do you prefer a different lead-in? Try: "I have some power here. In the best of all worlds I wish I had . . .", "My part of this was . . .", or "I regret that I . . ."

Anger can be so helpful

Anyone who has been harmed has anger. If we suppress anger, it turns into anxiety, depression, or numbness and fuels the drive to overeat. It is common for anger to be the "missing feeling" in the 3 Tool. Many of us have never seen healthy anger expressed or we experienced unsafe expressions of anger growing up. There is a positive side to anger, as it quickly reduces stress. A spark of anger unlocks the circuits that activate overeating. As you use EBT, your brain will learn how to use anger in a highly effective way. This takes practice, but before long, you will develop a healthy, safe, productive "A+ Anger" skill. This shift to using anger effectively is natural and universal – and it will happen for you in time.

I feel secure. Is that possible?

With so much stress overload, the thinking brain and emotional brain connection begins to wobble! Since this connection is the source of our security, we become anxious or tense. However, this tool reconnects the brain, and by using it you'll start to feel a sense of security. Your brain is connected!

Am I emotionally lopsided?

I hope so. We all are. The brain's processing starts with negative emotions because its primary role is keeping us from danger. Naturally, it goes right to the negative emotions. Only when the negative emotions have been felt and expressed does the brain enable you to access the positive emotions.

Positive emotions? They make me uncomfortable!

The reptilian brain favors negative emotions because they are most familiar, particularly when our set point is in stress. That will change with practice. Using this tool often is one of the most effective ways to feel comfortable with positive emotions.

I think I'm numb. Can this tool work for me?

Yes! Most of us are numb for good reason. If we do not have a full set of emotional tools, when we start to feel our feelings they will become stuck. They won't tell us what we need, only what we want. As you learn the tool, the brain becomes comfortable with emotions, and numbness fades.

Enjoy this tool and be aware that it will work sometimes and at other times feel rather flat. We're back where we started. The only way to make EBT really work for you is to keep laughing about the elusive and magical emotional brain! It's by experimenting with these tools that your brain changes!

Success Check Day 4

- **Daily Success**

  ☐ I continued my Joy Practice with 10 Check Ins and 10 Joy Points.

  ☐ I used the 3 Tool five or more times.

  ☐ I made one or more community connections for support with the 3 Tool.

- **Did I pass the Success Check? YES NO**

  If you did not pass, take another day to complete it, then move on.

- **My Amazing Learning:**

  _____

- **My Biggest Accomplishment:**

  _____

- **My Biggest Challenge:**

  _____

Well Done!

**You have completed Day 4 of The Joy Challenge.
Your next step is Day 5. Feel The Glow.**

Day 5. Feel the Glow

We are already on Day 5. Check to see if your reptilian brain is acting up yet. If you "accidentally" lost your book, that's the reptilian brain at work. Forgot to check in for two days? The reptile within protects how we fundamentally process life. When we make an upgrade in our emotional "software" it revolts and triggers stress and sabotage.

Keep your sense of humor. We're going to torment the reptilian brain even more today, because we will learn the tools for Brain States 1 and 2. These tools will take you to joy or deepen your joy.

The Brain State 1 Tool, the Compassion Tool, takes a momentarily great state and prolongs it. The Brain State 2 Tool, the Feelings Tool, takes an ordinary mood and turns it into a great mood that shuts off the desire to overeat.

As you feel connected, positive, loving, and creative at Brain State 1, watch for the reptilian brain to tell you that you should not feel that good, that it will never last, or that other people feel bad so that you should feel that bad or worse! Have a wonderful day learning these two amazing tools!

Why

The drive to overeat is very sensitive to stress. Even small stresses can trigger our Stress Circuits and drive us to eat when we aren't hungry. By being at Brain State 1, the Stress Circuits that drive overeating go offline. If we go the extra mile to spiral up to Brain State 1 often, our dopamine, oxytocin, and serotonin levels promote healthy eating naturally.

I have a robust lizard brain. I was the youngest in my family, and the older kids bullied me. Then I married a woman who did the same thing. It took two divorces to figure out I'm not an emotional punching bag. I never learned to be in joy. Joy to me was pizza, beer, tv, and texting, all at once. The 2 Tool gets me to Brain State 1. My lizard brain doesn't like that, but I do.

I'm taking this course so I can stuff myself with so many good feelings that I don't need to entertain myself with food. I want to get to Brain State 1 from Brain State 2. The more joy the better!

We're overcoming the drive to overeat and the reptile's desire to make us hold onto extra weight. We need an abundance of joy! It's essential to not put up with a measly Brain State 2. Make it to Brain State 1, even for a second, and it changes your body chemistry. Then use the 1 Tool to prolong that appetite-suppressing state!

These tools will spark a sense of connection within, a feeling of peace and power. They are quick and easy to use. In just 30 to 45 seconds, we can be at Brain State 1 or deepen that state!

I'm naturally compassionate when it comes to animals and anyone who is in need of some tenderness. I like feeling compassion. The 1 Tool works for me.

I didn't expect the 2 Tool to work so well. If I pause after saying, "How do I feel?" three feelings come to mind. I wait until two of them fade and the one strongest feeling becomes clear. Then I pause again. I ask myself, "What do I need?" Again, for about 20 seconds I have no idea what I need. Then some words appear in my mind. In that instant, I am at Brain State 1 and I haven't even asked the last question, nor have I met my supposed need. How strange!

How

The 1 Tool ("Compassion Tool") sustains Brain State 1. The surge of neurochemicals at Brain State 1 is better than the one triggered by eating ice cream. It is calorie-free and there is no food hangover.

With a bit of nudging from the words of the 1 Tool, our reward center lights up, and we feel elevated emotions. In that state of connection, our motivations are based on purpose. Our needs for safety, love, comfort, and pleasure are met and the healing chemicals of altruism fill the void and nourish our spirits.

The 1 Tool stops stress eating. We eat when we are hungry and get pleasure from food, but are so sensitive to our body's needs that eating when not hungry is not pleasurable. It does not feel good at all. That's the power of Brain State 1!

Basic emotions vs. elevated emotions

Basic emotions, such as feeling happy, lonely, or tired, are designed to alert us to our needs. When we are at the most connected state, Brain State 1, we do not have needs. Our "need" is to feel the emotions of connection: love, compassion, gratitude, hope, forgiveness, awe, and joy.

The 1 Tool – Compassion Tool
• Feel compassion for myself.
• Feel compassion for others.
• Feel compassion for all living beings.

The purpose of the 1 Tool is to prolong and deepen our elevated emotions. Each of the three lead-ins is a "command" to yourself to feel the elevated emotion of compassion. First, you instruct yourself to feel compassion for yourself.

Pause to feel your compassion . . .

Then you pause for a moment and notice a wave of compassion in your body. That body sensation confirms that you are at Brain State 1 and encourages you to continue using the tool to experience an even stronger natural high.

Next, you tell yourself to feel compassion for others. Once you feel in your body that wave of compassion for others, you are ready for the last command of the tool. You tell yourself to extend your compassion to all living beings. When you do that, the drive to overeat will vanish. With that final emotional flourish, pause and feel a glow.

Where did my compassion go?

You are a compassionate person. When you are connected, it is easy to feel compassion for yourself and others! However, when you are in stress, compassion vanishes. This can be disconcerting, because right when we are convinced we are a nice person, we turn judgmental, rigid, and unkind. It's really important to know that if compassion does not flow, it's not our fault.

Those Stress Circuits that trigger the cortisol cascade block our natural capacity for kindness, love, and compassion. The problem is not us. It's a wire that triggers a stressed brain state. Before long, we'll start frying those wires!

Why cortisol matters!

Cortisol is the main stress hormone
and "public health enemy #1,"
as it switches on the Stress Triangle.

"I use the EBT tools to shut off cortisol."

The 2 Tool (the "Feelings Tool")

Use the 2 Tool when you feel present and aware, but lack that certain glow of feeling rewarded. When we are at Brain State 1, our emotions accurately signal us to meet our true needs. This tool guides our way and lands us back at Brain State 1, activating the drive to eat healthy.

This tool is miraculous. By the time I ask the first two questions, I'm connected, present, and in the flow. I tingle with warmth and excitement about . . . being alive and having a chance to figure out what my dreams are, and how to make them come true!

The 2 Tool – Feelings Tool

- How do I feel?
- What do I need?
- Do I need support?

How do I feel?

The trick to making this tool amazingly effective is to ask the question, "How do I feel?" and then pause. Several emotions will compete for dominance. Pause!

After about 10 to 20 seconds, one emotion will be strongest. Based on evolutionary biology, the strongest feeling points to the most important need. Knowing what we need is so essential to our survival that we experience a surge of dopamine from being aware of our need! We are at Brain State 1 before taking any action to meet our identified need.

To identify your need, ask, "What do I need?" In other words, given that feeling, what is the corresponding need? Pause until some words appear in your mind, then ask yourself, "Do I need support?" Check whether or not you need support from others to meet that need. Sometimes you will and sometimes you will not.

Basic Feelings

		Negative		
angry	sad	afraid	guilty	tired
tense	hungry	full	lonely	sick
		Positive		
grateful	happy	secure	proud	rested
relaxed	satisfied	loved	loving	healthy

Being at Brain State 2 is good for me. Mostly, I'm at 3 or 4. I asked myself, "How do I feel?" I wasn't sure, and then sadness came up. I had no idea I was sad. Okay, I'm sad. What do I do with my sadness? I asked myself, "What do I need?" The answer was that I need to feel my feelings and let them fade. When I said those words to myself, instantly I was at Brain State 1. Do I need support? The answer was no. I was already at Brain State 1.

What do I need? The logical need vs. the intuitive need

Sometimes our need is very logical. I am hungry. I need to eat. However, most of the time it is not logical. All needs are relative. If we overuse the thinking brain to try to "figure out" what we need, we cause rumination, anxiety, and stress!

We can ask the question in a deeper way, piercing the veil of logic and entering into the wisdom of the emotional brain. When we ask the question, "What do I need?" and pause for long enough (usually about 10 to 20 seconds), words that convey the accurate need will arrive in our mind.

All you did differently was to trust your body, trust the tools, and do the hardest thing of all – tolerate not knowing, just for a few seconds.

The primitive emotional brain will process all that information for you and come up with information about what you need, and then spiral you up to Brain State 1. The survival of the species is based on using our whole brain, not just the thinking brain. When we engage in that process, we often experience a surge of dopamine – the generous reward of evolutionary biology. This has major implications for stress eating. When you use this tool to get to a strong Brain State 1, chances are that you will feel so rewarded that you will not have a drive to overeat.

I wasn't stressed at all. Perhaps bored, and I had an ache in my neck from too many hours of word processing. Normally I would have taken a restroom break and found something to eat, but I used a tool. I asked, "How do I feel?" I wasn't sure, but after a bit, the word "lonely" appeared in my mind. I pondered that for a few moments, then I asked myself, "What do I need?" The answer appeared in my mind, too. It was to appreciate that my job was pretty lonely and to have compassion for myself. I felt the glow and lost all interest in food. Did I need support? No, I was at ONE.

By pausing for long enough to discover our deeper, intuitive need, we often go against the logical need. For example, if we want to release weight for the deeper need of vibrancy or freedom, slight experiences of hunger feel good to us.

I was taught to eat everything on my plate. If food was in front of me, my job was to eat it. There wasn't anything intuitive about eating. So I said to myself, "How do I feel? I feel hungry. What do I need?" Logically, I knew that I needed food, but I paused for a few moments. I asked myself the question again. "What do I really need? I need to have a glass of water and see if my hunger goes away. I want to lose weight and that makes feeling slightly hungry nurturing to me."

Do I need support from others?

The last question of this tool checks whether or not we need assistance from others. The emotional brain is a lonely brain. We must connect emotionally to the deepest part of ourselves and that allows us to be vulnerable enough to ask for support from others. It is that giving and receiving of support and love that shuts off stress eating. We cannot isolate without activating stress eating or other addictions. When in doubt, ask for support!

Now you have the brain-based resiliency tools that work for the higher brain states. The 1 Tool and 2 Tool are so powerful. Practice using these tools many times today and notice how easy it is to be at Brain State 1. You'll be feasting on natural pleasures and find that you could care less about overeating. Enjoy experimenting with these tools!

Success Check Day 5

● **Daily Success**

☐ I continued my Joy Practice with 10 Check Ins and 10 Joy Points.

☐ I tried the 1 Tool and the 2 Tool at least three times each.

☐ I made one or more community connections for support with these tools.

● **Did I pass the Success Check?   YES   NO**

If you did not, stay with this activity for one more day, then move on.

● **My Amazing Learning:**

_____

● **My Biggest Accomplishment:**

_____

● **My Biggest Challenge:**

_____

Congratulations!

**You have completed Day 5 of The Joy Challenge.
Your next step is Day 6. Cycle Tool.**

Day 6. Cycle Tool

Today may be the most important day for you in this course. You'll learn how to use a trio of tools that enable you to discover that hidden brain pathway from stress to joy, so that throughout the day, you can use your own brain to activate that glow.

This is a time to cut loose and have a lot of fun with these tools. It's so strange to think that stating a few words, then pausing to notice what words bubble up from your unconscious mind, then going on to the next set of words and another pause, can change your drive to overeat, your tendency to gain weight, and the chemicals in every cell of your body. However, once you experience even a slight shift in your body from using the tools, chances are you'll want to use the tools and feel that way again!

Why

We use the Cycle Tool to shut off the Stress Circuits and short-circuit the wires that cause stress eating. Also, it's a great tool to use for everyday stress, as no matter what wire is triggering us to be at Brain State 4, the Cycle Tool will spiral us up to Brain State 1.

Later on, you'll use this tool to focus on the precise eating style and wire that bother you the most. You'll use it in a deeper way to transform an old wire that causes stress into a new one that activates joy. You'll use it to reconsolidate the overeating wire, turning it into a healthy eating wire. Right now, the challenge is to become comfortable using this tool in the simplest way. Much the way you learned how to guess your brain state, having fun with it, now you'll have fun learning the Cycle Tool.

There are three variations of the Cycle Tool. To determine which tool you want to use, check the benefit that you want. If you want to have more positive emotions, choose the Be Positive Tool. If you want to feel better, perhaps you are feeling tense, stuck, or lost, use the Feel Better Tool. If you feel triggered and have cravings, knee-jerk overreactions, or keep repeating the same behavior even though it doesn't work for you, use the Stop a Trigger Tool.

The Best Brain State of All

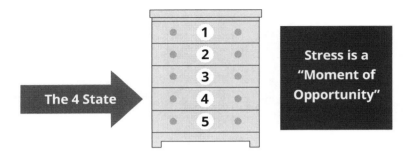

The 4 State → [dresser drawers 1, 2, 3, 4, 5]

Stress is a "Moment of Opportunity"

Stress is a moment of opportunity!

As you use this tool, you'll probably notice that you feel better quickly. The experience of being stressed, then using a technique that in two to four minutes gives you an amazing insight and a natural high, can be thrilling.

Not only can that "spiral up" feel great, but we need stress to unlock the old circuit. Without a brief spark of stress, the wiring seems to change, but when a stressful experience occurs, the old pattern comes back. For example, we eat healthy and lose weight, then stress comes along and that old stress eating circuit returns. At Brain State 3, we're not stressed enough to unlock faulty circuits and at Brain State 5, the thinking brain isn't functional enough to use the Cycle Tool. In this way, Brain State 4 gives us what we need to change rapidly and in profound ways.

How

All Cycles start with a complaint, talking about what bothers you. When we are at Brain State 4, we need the prefrontal cortex (the internalized good parent) to take charge. Stating what is bothering us accomplishes that, but what follows is some emotional processing. If the stress is situational and there is no strong circuit causing stress overload, then expressing feelings is all that is needed. If stress is ramping up because an old wire is being activated, then we can use expressing emotions to discover that circuit, and begin to rewire it.

Play with the Cycle Tool!

- **Be Positive Cycle** – Switch off negative emotions and activate positive emotions

- **Feel Better Cycle** – Stop feeling bad, lost, abandoned, tense, or upset and feel (much) better

- **Stop a Trigger Cycle** – Quiet the drive to repeat old patterns and overreact, and encode new patterns and balanced responses

---

- **Be Positive Cycle**
  Clear stress and negative emotions and positive ones arise.

- **Feel Better Cycle**
  Discover and change a false generalization, such as "I do not have power" or "I am not worthy."

- **Stop a Trigger Cycle**
  Discover and change a false association, such as "I get my love from food."

Like the other tools, the trick is to use your neocortex to state the lead-in, then pause, and wait for words to bubble up to your conscious mind. Feel the feelings. Then go on to the next lead-in.

Experiment!

Check In, Select 4   ### Try out a Tool

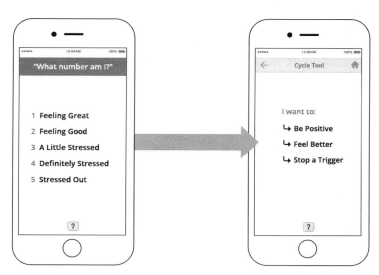

I was raised with shame, I don't want to express guilt

How do we discover wires? By stating what we believe we could have done differently. We complete the phrase: *I feel guilty that . . .* And if we state what we truly believe we could have done differently, we discover that we did that because of a wire. That guilt draws us right to the wire (the unreasonable expectation) that is the problem, so we can rewire it.

I don't like to be angry

The anger we use in the Cycle Tool is not the kind of anger people express when they yell at someone or go into a rage. It is a very carefully constructed expression of anger that is a protest against being hurt. As soon as you activate the reptilian brain and express enough anger to unlock the circuit, the anger goes away. It flows into feelings that heal. Anger has a unique role in activating circuits so that we can rewire them. It is the only negative emotion that is associated with power. Start slowly and practice safe, effective A+ Anger. Go at your own pace. In time you will have a great A+ Anger skill, and you'll be crushing circuits right and left!

All cycles begin the same way

Although all three Cycles start out with the same lead-ins, they each finish off differently in order to meet your need. However, each of the cycles reduces stress and activates positive emotions, so you cannot go wrong! Let's look at the first part of one Cycle, then complete it in each of the three ways.

All Cycles Begin the Same Way

- **Focus on what is bothering you**
  The situation is . . .
  > (COMPLAIN: STATE FACTS, NOT FEELINGS)
  What I'm most stressed about is . . .
  > (ONE SIMPLE STATEMENT, ABOUT ONE TOPIC)

- **Express anger (A+ Anger) to unlock the circuit**
  I feel angry that . . .
  I can't stand it that . . .
  I hate it that . . .
  > (plus more anger until your mind shuts off)

- **Feel your feelings (pause before and after each feeling)**
  I feel sad that . . .
  I feel afraid that . . .
  I feel guilty that . . .

Example of how all Cycles begin the same way

The situation is . . . I am tired of overeating and I don't know what to do about it. Right now I feel like getting a donut or some cookies. What I'm most stressed about is . . . I want something I should not have. I feel angry that . . . I can't have it. I can't stand it that . . . I want sugar but I have to limit myself. I HATE it that . . . I can't have what I want when I want it!!! I hate that!!! I feel sad that . . . I need food so much. I feel afraid that . . . there is something wrong with me. I feel guilty that . . . I don't just eat the sugar and stop worrying about it!

The Be Positive Cycle

Use this Cycle Tool when you notice yourself being negative and quite stressed. The allostatic circuit itself is not causing the negativity, but the stimuli from your body, brain, and external environment are ramping up your stress. Be sure to complain a lot and express plenty of anger. However, after that, negative feelings will melt away and positive emotions will flow. You'll be back to glow. This is a wonderful tool that you may end up using many times each day.

The Be Positive Cycle
• I feel grateful that . . . I am learning not to judge myself.   • I feel happy that . . . I am doing something about my overeating.   • I feel secure that . . . I am changing.   • I feel proud that . . . I am trying something new.

The Feel Better Cycle

Use this Cycle Tool when you feel stressed or bad, but not triggered. The circuits that this tool deactivates are basic expectations or core circuits that were encoded by stressful experiences long ago. They are false generalizations, sending ineffective messages that arose in the moment that the brain misencoded as true. For instance, in a moment when we felt like we did not matter, a persistent and incontestable message was encoded: I do not matter. These are horrendous wires, and rewiring them is the foundation for advanced training in the method, but you can start to "loosen" them up now. The core unreasonable expectations to watch for when you use this Cycle Tool are: I do not matter. I am bad. I have to be perfect. I do not have power. I do not exist. I cannot do good. I am not worthy. I cannot have joy. These wires activate the Stress Triangle chronically, draining our neurotransmitters and causing not only chronic stress, but inflammation. These messages can make us feel bad enough that the brain triggers an escape, a brain glitch, such as a strong drive to overeat. Let's see how using the Feel Better Cycle tool completes this Cycle:

The Feel Better Cycle
OF COURSE I did that, because my unreasonable expectation is . . . (example: I do not have power.) Grind it in (3 to 6 times each): SLOW — I . . . DO . . . have . . . power. RAMP UP — That's ridiculous. I DO have power! JOY — I DO HAVE POWER and I'm going to use it!

OF COURSE I wouldn't just eat the sugar and stop worrying about it, because my unreasonable expectation is . . . I must be perfect. Oh, that rings so true. My unreasonable expectation is that I must be perfect. I want to change that wire! I . . . do . . . NOT . . . have . . . to . . . be . . . PERFECT. I . . . do . . . not . . . have . . . to . . . be . . . perfect. I do not have to be perfect. That's ridiculous. I don't have to be perfect. How ridiculous is that? I just need to be who I am. I just need to be who I really am. I just need to be who I am!!!

The Stop a Trigger Cycle

Use the Stop a Trigger Cycle Tool to short-circuit a response that triggers an unstoppable drive. These circuits are encoded during moments of stress overload in which the brain "crosses wires." They launch a fight-or-flight response and tell us we are going to die if we do not escape. That ridiculous response which does not meet our needs, but was a quick fix in the moment, is now stored in the least plastic area of our brain. That response is now activated by even small stresses during daily life. By using the Cycle Tool, the unconscious message becomes conscious so the thinking brain can assess it and change it. What's more, because of the liberal release of emotions that preceded the discovery, the thinking brain is functioning better and appreciates that getting love from sugar is not that effective!

The Stop a Trigger Cycle
OF COURSE I did that, because my unreasonable expectation is . . . (example: I get my safety from food.) Grind it in (3 to 6 times each): SLOW — I . . . can . . . NOT . . . get . . . safety . . . from . . . FOOD. RAMP UP — That's ridiculous. I can NOT get SAFETY from food! JOY — I get my safety from inside me!

This false message can trigger the Stress Triangle, and symptoms that bother us, such as unhealthy behaviors, negative moods, and disturbing or repetitive thoughts. They are unconscious and extremely strong. When we shut off these circuits by doing a Cycle, the drive to repeat the old pattern shuts down for the moment. We are in control again. Let's complete our sample Cycle with the Stop a Trigger Cycle tool:

OF COURSE I wouldn't just eat the sugar and stop worrying about it, because my unreasonable expectation is . . . I get my safety from . . . sugar. No, that doesn't ring true. Let me try it again. OF COURSE I wouldn't just eat the sugar and stop worrying about it, because I get my . . . security from . . . eating sweets. Yes, that's right! I can NOT . . . get my SECURITY . . . from eating . . . sweets. I can NOT . . . get . . . my . . . security . . . from . . . eating . . . sweets. No I can't. I can NOT get my security from eating sweets. That's ridiculous. I can NOT get security from sweets. That will never work. I get my security from connecting to the deepest part of myself and feeling good about myself no matter what. I get my security from connecting to myself and loving myself. I get my security from connecting to myself and loving ME!

By using this tool, we can shut off the drive to overeat for the moment, and avoid overeating much of the time. We can not only deactivate the Stress Triangle, but step out of the stress eating cycle.

They are at One, and they have a new plan that's reasonable and brings them a surge of joy.

No matter which Cycle tool you select, you can benefit your brain and feel better.

Take Purposeful Action
When the Cycle Tool returns you to joy, sometimes you are so charged up that you know precisely what to do and why you are doing it. You have already faced whatever essential pain of life you need to accept and in your mind's eye is the prize. Your brain is already joyfully anticipating your amazing reward for following through.

The Take Action Tool
• I expect myself to do the best I can to . . .
• My positive, powerful thought . . .
• The essential pain is . . .
• My earned reward is . . .

Whenever that is not the case, it's essential to tack onto your Cycle the Take Action Tool. By doing this you become passionate and are purpose-driven. Just state what you expect of yourself. Always it's to do the best you can and no better. That last little bit of personal punishment, that rigid, unloving perfectionism, typically harms relationships, spiritual connection, and health. Who needs that?

Next fortify yourself with some encouraging words, like "I can do that!" or "That matters to me!" This gives your brain enough time to bring up an image of you following through. When that image appears, you can identify the hard part of following through. That essential pain of life is the best medicine, because if you can accept that, you will be aware of the higher-order reason for taking that action. A Joy Point naturally follows and you are on your way . . . passionate, purposeful, and redefining what is possible. You are creating joy in your life!

I expect myself to do the best I can to . . . get some sleep. My positive, powerful thought? That's important to me. The essential pain? I am not in complete control. My reward is . . . vibrancy.

No more blaming ourselves

The Cycle Tool can rapidly clear away our tendency to blame ourselves or be confused about why we do what we do. We do what the unconscious mind tells us to do. Whenever things aren't going well, and you are lucky enough to be at Brain State 4, do a Cycle. You'll discover the circuit, and a glow will come over your face. It's not your fault! What's more, you can change the unconscious expectation, so you'll be less likely to repeat that pattern. This is a level of personal power that most of us dream of and never have. You now have it!

Easy does it!

Start experimenting and playing with these tools. Try a tool. If it doesn't work, try another tool. Each use of the tool impacts your brain, both learning what works and learning what does not work. Each try at doing a Cycle is productive in its own way.

The Cycles you do today are quick and easy. Move through the lead-ins rapidly to relieve stress or cravings. We call them "Quick and Easy Cycles." They are fast passes at using the tool, using the lead-ins and noticing what words bubble up. The entire Cycle takes one to four minutes and is somewhat messy, particularly at first.

For best results, be sure that your Cycles are fun to do. Are you the kind of person who has fun only when you are confronting the reptilian brain? If so, experiment with making this fun by doing a Triple Cycle, using all three types of Cycles, one right after the other. Start with the Be Positive Cycle, then use the Feel Better Cycle Tool. Last, use the Stop a Trigger Cycle. Chances are, you'll learn a lot and, by the time you complete all three, you'll feel absolutely great!

Right now we are using the Cycle Tool for immediate results. Later, starting on Day 9, we'll use this tool in an intensive way to rewire circuits for more lasting results.

For now, focus on being breezy in using this tool, and have a glorious time discovering your power to switch off wires in your unconscious mind!

Success Check Day 6

- **Daily Success**

☐ I continued my Joy Practice with 10 Check Ins and 10 Joy Points.

☐ I tried each of the three Cycle Tools at least once.

☐ I made one or more community connections for support with doing Cycles.

- **Did I pass the Success Check?   YES   NO**

If you did not, stay with this activity for one more day, then move on.

- **My Amazing Learning:**

_____

- **My Biggest Accomplishment:**

_____

- **My Biggest Challenge:**

_____

Congratulations!

You have completed Day 6 of The Joy Challenge.
Your next step is Day 7. Damage Control Tool.

Day 7. Damage Control Tool

You're checking in, scoring Joy Points, and perhaps feeling a bit happier. You have been giving your brain a workout, asking it to connect in new ways, staying present in the moment, feeling your feelings, and spiraling up!

You and those around you like that! However, buried at the bottom of the brain, the reptile within is not happy. It does not like you disengaging from stress and starting to become wired for joy. Your inner lizard is apt to become irritable, as it likes your old set point in stress and attaching to food for safety, love, comfort, and pleasure, even though you are not hungry.

Having no capacity to speak, the reptilian brain spews stress chemicals and triggers a Brain State 5 – sometimes a big one! We can't have that. We can use our neocortex, our internal overseer, to quiet the reptile. It is not happy, so we use our power to calm it down.

Today's skill, the Damage Control Tool, gives you the power to keep that reptile from triggering chronic stress.

Why

We use our power to control the reptilian brain because if we are passive and let it take charge, the Stress Triangle causes cravings, hunger, lethargy, and weight gain. We have the capacity to

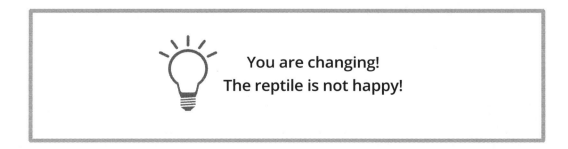

You are changing!
The reptile is not happy!

stop the stress center (amygdala) from getting that whole process activated and then causing the stress buzzer to get stuck on, so let's use it.

We have a great deal of power to do that because the original stress – an upset family member or having a barrage of self-doubt – is not the problem. It's the secondary stress that harms us. It can be that we "catch" another person's stress, become stressed about being stressed, or have come to believe that we are powerless to tame the reptile. That's what harms us, and that is what we fix by using the Damage Control Tool.

How

The Damage Control Tool involves a series of statements that help us connect to ourselves and calm the reptile within. These same statements are core to all major world religions.

We appreciate that the problem is not us, but these wires and the chemicals they activate. We understand that raising our set point is very threatening to the reptile. The happier you become, the more it becomes touchy, snappish, and insecure. It will continue to act up periodically, and we must be the kind but strong parent and help it calm down. Always assume that the reptile is pulling out all the stops and activating a full-blown stress response. Use body movements first, then tell yourself: Do not judge. Minimize harm. Know it will pass.

Start with the Full Blown Damage Control Tool, (the 5 Plus Tool), using simple, rhythmic activities that work well to stop stress overload. Belly breathing is evidence-based for reducing physiologic stress. Just turn your attention to your body and focus on your breathing. Watch your belly move up and down and be sure to use a long, slow exhale. Do something rhythmic that you would do to calm an infant, such as rocking in your chair, stroking your arm, or rubbing your neck.

Let's make the reptile a bit happier:
The Damage Control Tool

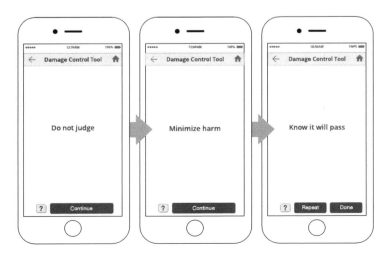

When you feel a bit better, use the regular Damage Control Tool on your own or by using the app. Repeat the statements: Do not judge. Minimize harm. Know it will pass. Do this in whatever style works for you – slow or fast. Don't hold back with repeating the words. Sometimes it takes 10 to 30 repetitions of this tool to calm a circuit.

The 5 Tools

The 5 PLUS Tool – (Full Blown Damage Control)
- Rocking back and forth
- Belly breathing
- Stroking the body

The 5 Tool – (Damage Control)
- Do not judge
- Minimize harm
- Know it will pass

What do the words of Damage Control mean?

The first phrase of the Damage Control Tool is *Do Not Judge*. It is normal to judge ourselves or others when we are in stress overload. It's cortisol that makes us do it. You might notice that you tend to do one or the other. A person who distances tends to judge others. A person who merges tends to judge themselves. You can revise the words to say either of these statements or both of them, such as to say, "Do not judge. I will not judge myself." or "Do not judge. I will not judge others. I will not judge myself!" Feel free to personalize this tool.

What does *Minimize harm* mean? Don't we mean do no harm? The neurophysiology of stress ensures that there will be harm. The stress overload alone impacts every organ system in significant and deleterious ways. In addition, in the 5 State, our thinking brain is offline, and we lose our good judgment, flexible thinking, and impulse control.

The minimize harm statement means that we accept that this is a harmful state, but we are going to do our best to control the damage. Perhaps we will eat a large bite of dark chocolate, down a diet soda, or sprinkle cinnamon sugar on apple slices. Some people sense that they have a "mega-circuit" so that even a tiny bit of a substance triggers unstoppable drives. The instruction to minimize harm won't work for them. They prefer abstinence. If abstinence is your goal, you may want to personalize your Damage Control statement and choose words such as "do not eat sugar" or "no comfort foods." Always personalize the tools to meet your needs!

What about the phrase *Know it will pass*? The statement is general because depending on the strength and dominance of the circuit, a Brain State 5 can persist for quite a while. The allostatic circuits are positive feedback loops, which means they have no shut-off valves. If they are triggered, they can trigger other circuits that were encoded at the same level of stress. However, the state – sooner or later – does pass! We use this statement to remind ourselves that it won't last forever!

When we are at 5,
faulty messages ring true

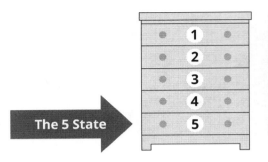

The 5 State

Examples
- **I must be perfect.**
- **I am bad if I overeat.**
- **I am not worthy.**
- **I have no power.**

Worst of all, because this is the "survival circuit" drawer, these messages are extremely convincing. The survival of the species is based on our believing and obeying the messages in the 5th Drawer reflexively. We believe these messages, and each one stresses us out even more. The result? We can be stuck in Brain State 5 for hours, days, or even weeks! In that state, impulse control vanishes and reflexive ("knee-jerk") responses rule us. Most people have no idea how to short-circuit a 5 State. This is why using the 5 PLUS Tool as your first defense and the 5 Tool right after that are core life skills. Everyone goes to 5 and everyone needs a personalized process for calming the reptile within!

Protect Yourself from Brain State 5

- Use the 5 PLUS Tool as your first defense.
- The prefrontal cortex is offline – be careful!
- Stress causes a time warp – know it will pass!

Going to 5 then spiraling up to 1 is core to the human experience

Brain State 5 never feels good! However, our repeated dips into Brain State 5, and the rise to Brain State 1 that follows, are core to human development. The 5 State is woven into our lives as a way of helping us evolve and update our brain's emotional architecture. Every moment at Brain State 5 triggers the reptile. It activates the family of circuits in our 5th Drawer and if we use the tools, those circuits quiet down and we update our brain and can even spiral up to Brain State 1.

I am grateful to know that the problem is the reptile, because when I'm at Brain State 5, I'm sure there is something wrong with me. I go to the store and find the absolute worst foods I can get. I have been letting my lizard control me, and the idea that I can sweet talk it is appealing. I can do that!

The light side of Brain State 5

What follows a moment at Brain State 5 is often a natural high one can experience in no other way. The astonishing spiral ups after stress overload can bring about a very strong and healing Brain State 1 PLUS!

The "joy" of Brain State 5 can happen in two ways. Sometimes a Brain State 5 seemingly miraculously turns into a Brain State 1. If we stay present to our feelings when we feel horrible, something good can happen. Perhaps we surrender to the greater good or discover some kernel of wisdom in the experience. At other times we use the tools to spiral up back to One.

I have my life so well-organized that I almost never go to Brain State 5. I was not sure how I was going to do this activity. Then my sister was diagnosed with cancer and I went right to the 5 State. I did the breathing and brought a kind heart to my reptile. Perhaps love is the key ingredient here. I spiraled up to Brain State 1. I'm not sure how that happened, but it was life-changing for me.

The other joy of Brain State 5 is that stress offers a moment of opportunity to rewire faulty circuits. Only when we are in highly stressed states are our wires unlocked so that we can transform them. The problem is that it's hard to dislodge ourselves from that state. It's not the "primary stress" of being triggered that harms us, but the "secondary stress" of staying at Brain State 5.

The Perfection of Brain State 5
• A moment of opportunity
• A prelude to Brain State 1
• A time for profound connection

I know my reptile is prickly. I don't tell anyone my hopeless, dark thoughts that come up at Brain State 5. I'm using my 5 moments to test how much I love myself. If I can go deeper inside then and love myself, that could change my relationship with myself. That would definitely help stop my overeating.

When in the emotional crisis of a 5 State, we are in the middle of a fight-or-flight response that tells us that there is no hope, and all is lost. It is not. Instead, if we can find a shred of compassion for ourselves, any semblance of loving connection, we can change our brain for the better.

Experiment with this tool and personalize it. The reptile is not happy that you are happy, but by soothing it a bit, you'll feel more peace and power from within.

Success Check Day 7

- **Daily Success**

☐ I continued my Joy Practice with 10 Check Ins and 10 Joy Points.

☐ I used the 5 Tool and the 5 PLUS Tool three times each (even if I was not actually at Brain State 5).

☐ I made one or more community connections for support with these tools.

- **Did I pass the Success Check?   YES   NO**

If you did not, stay with this activity for one more day, then move on.

- **My Amazing Learning:**

_____

- **My Biggest Accomplishment:**

_____

- **My Biggest Challenge:**

_____

Congratulations!

You have completed Day 7 of The Joy Challenge.
Your next step is Day 8. Lifestyle Reset #1 Exercise.

Day 8. Lifestyle Reset #1 Exercise

Congratulations on completing Spiral Up to Joy! Now you can use EBT to switch off overeating circuits and activate healthy eating circuits. You can use your prefrontal cortex (neocortex) to change your experience of life in the moment. You can do that!

As you acquire new skills, you will ease stress and feel more rewarded through gradually making lifestyle changes in the form of five small but important resets. By taking it in small "chunks" of change, the reptilian brain is less likely to be triggered.

When you complete all five lifestyle resets and learn more about the tools, you'll have a culminating experience of personalizing your lifestyle to maximize vibrancy. Then you'll train the brain's habit center (basal ganglia) in that lifestyle as you continue with the program and become wired for joy. There are six resets in this program. The first lifestyle reset is to exercise.

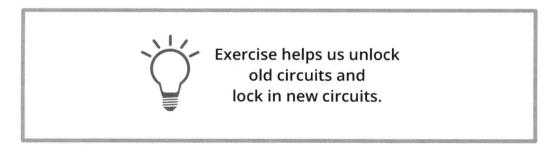

Exercise helps us unlock
old circuits and
lock in new circuits.

Why

The strategy is to start by moving your body and feeling the joy of honoring the sensations and emotions that arise when you move. Moving reduces stress. Any kind of moving counts, even standing up and swinging your arms in circles or doing a little dance in place!

Exercise boosts a chemical that helps change the brain. BDNF (Brain-derived neurotrophic factor) increases when we exercise, and the combination of BDNF and intensive learning generates new neurons and locks them into our wiring. The brain changes more rapidly. Imagine old circuits that blocked your joy giving way to new circuits that amplify it.

Why BDNF matters!

Brain-derived neurotrophic factor is "miracle grow" for neurons.
Thirty minutes per day of exercise using major muscle groups
(legs and arms) increases BDNF synthesis by 300%.

"I exercise for optimal brain health."

The idea of exercising doesn't appeal to me, but if it helps me rewire my binge eating sooner, then I'll do it. Maybe I'll warm up in the sauna, then listen to my favorite tunes while I work out. That sounds fun!

Move for 30 minutes each day, plus be active!

Move for 30 minutes or more each day. Choose activities that use your major muscle groups, such as walking, dancing, hiking, or playing sports. If you are not able to do these things, start by standing up, bending your knees, stretching, or moving your arms in some way that feels good (and fun!) to you. This core lifestyle tool of being more active and moving in joy increases your flexibility, strength, and endurance. You build a better brain as you enjoy your body and your life.

Why do you need to have fun for your exercise to count? Exercise that is stressful does not improve neuroplasticity. The best exercise prescription is to do something you like, that is fun for you, and to do it throughout the day. For instance, a few minutes here and there of walking, climbing stairs, or stretching all count.

The Move In Joy Prescription

- Instead of sitting, STAND.
- Instead of standing, MOVE.
- Always make it FUN!

How

Now that your exercise prescription is to have fun while moving, start experimenting. Read the list of activities on the next page and check off all the ones that sound like fun to you. Try them until you have at least three activities you enjoy!

Exercise in Joy Checklist

- ☐ Turn on your favorite music and rock out at home.
- ☐ Does a co-worker want to meet? Suggest a walk and talk!
- ☐ Try solo stretching, relaxation, or yoga.
- ☐ Take a walk at lunchtime and listen to music.
- ☐ Play a sport: tennis, golf, baseball, volleyball . . .
- ☐ Locate a basketball court and shoot hoops.
- ☐ Play hide and seek with kids (or adults).
- ☐ Take the stairs.
- ☐ Find a happy gym with many ways to be playful.
- ☐ Give your partner or spouse a vigorous massage.
- ☐ Enjoy walking meditation or prayer.
- ☐ Sign up for classes in your favorite martial art.
- ☐ Take the dog for a walk, play Frisbee or fetch.
- ☐ Go outside in the morning: walk and watch the sunrise.
- ☐ Invite your romantic partner to exercise with you – be creative!
- ☐ Take a five-minute stretch break at work.
- ☐ Bike to and from work or the store.
- ☐ Get going with projects: cleaning, painting, gardening, building . . .
- ☐ Dance with your children, spouse, partner, or friend.
- ☐ Use a standing desk and isolate muscle groups as you write.
- ☐ Join a roller derby league or soccer team.
- ☐ Play a musical instrument like a violin or guitar standing up.
- ☐ Go for a morning swim at the local pool.
- ☐ Take a walk at twilight and enjoy the night air and magical light.
- ☐ Invite a friend to walk or run with you.

Success Check Day 8

- **Daily Success**

  ☐ I continued my Joy Practice with 10 Check Ins and 10 Joy Points.

  ☐ I reset my lifestyle to move in joy (including 30 minutes of exercise).

  ☐ I made one or more community connections for support with my lifestyle reset.

- **Did I pass the Success Check?   YES   NO**

  If you did not, stay with this activity for one more day, then move on.

- **My Amazing Learning:**

  _____

- **My Biggest Accomplishment:**

  _____

- **My Biggest Challenge:**

  _____

Congratulations!

You have completed Day 8 of The Joy Challenge.
Your next step is Day 9. Discover Your Food Circuit.

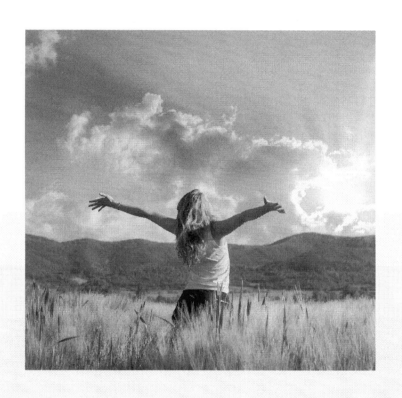

Eat Healthy

Day 9. Discover Your Food Circuit

We are now moving into the most exciting part of the book: rewiring circuits!

We'll start with the drive to overeat. In the next three days, you'll develop a Power Grind In for Food. This is a personalized tool that short-circuits cravings and transforms your Food Circuit. It changes that wire into a pathway that causes you to meet your needs and activates a desire to eat healthy.

Then, after a day of resetting our lifestyle, we'll take three days to develop a Power Grind In for Mood. All overeating is rooted in a stressed mood. By rewiring the drive for that emotional state, your Food Circuit will be easier to rewire.

Later in the program, focus on activating the drive to release weight by rewiring the Love Circuit (decreasing relationship stress that can fuel overeating) and the Body Circuit (making peace with our body to enhance our desire to release weight).

The Food Circuit

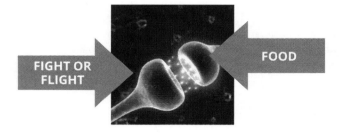

Why

Our Food Circuit creates hunger, cravings, and lethargy. The circuit itself is a "fight-or-flight" wire. It may not seem to be strong, but it is. The cascade of stress chemicals it unleashes causes the thinking brain and emotional brain to disconnect. Without neural integration (a connected brain), we do not have access to the emotional and sensory information to develop a healthy relationship with food. Our hunger signals are misguided and it's harder to know what we need. The disconnected brain is so judgmental! And all-or-nothing thinking takes over. No wonder we overeat! Once you clear this circuit, your natural capacity to eat when you are hungry, stop when you are satisfied, and enjoy your food (even more!) will kick in.

This is why we will discover, negate, and ultimately transform this Food Circuit, using the three-day rewiring plan. After using this plan, we will have a Power Grind In for Food. It is a series of statements that you can use to stop cravings, and over time, break the old Food Circuit and encode a new circuit that instructs you to listen to and honor your body's needs. You can eat only when hungry, eat healthy food, or eat in whatever way that meets your needs.

Instead of being stuck in the stress eating cycle, you will step out of it and find yourself eating healthy naturally. It will not be hard because you will have addressed the root cause of your stress eating: your wiring.

How

For each of the four major circuits you will discover in this book, you will use the same rewiring process. There are three steps: discover, negate, and transform. Take one step per day. If you need more time for a step, it is important to take that time!

The EBT 3-Day Rewiring Plan

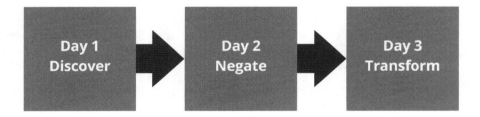

Circuits vary in intensity

Circuits can be encoded in any brain state. Eating for purpose is healthy eating. No rewiring needed! However, stress eating is eating when we are not hungry for emotional purposes: safety, love, comfort, or pleasure. The more stressed our state, the stronger the drive to overeat.

Day 1. Discover your Circuit

Begin by discovering the specific circuit you want to rewire. You'll do that today for your Food Circuit. It involves using the Stop a Trigger Cycle Tool to complain about whatever it is about overeating that bothers you the most. The result is that you activate and unlock the circuit so that you can update it.

Day 2. Negate your Circuit

Next, weaken the circuit. Just the way that one must make a left turn in a car before continuing the arc to make a U-turn, changing a circuit requires steps. A quick hairpin turn of expectations triggers the reptilian brain, and in stress overload, the rewiring process shuts down. You'll negate the circuit, that is, add the word "NOT" to the unreasonable expectation. For example, if the unreasonable expectation is, "I get my safety from overeating," the negated statement is, "I can NOT get my safety from overeating."

Day 3. Transform your Circuit

During the last day, you'll create a new circuit, one that tells you to connect with yourself, use a new approach to this stressor, and bring to mind a higher-order reward. This completes your Power Grind In and you can start using it four times daily to rewire the circuit.

The EBT 3-Day Rewiring Plan

- Day 1. Discover your Circuit
- Day 2. Negate your Circuit
- Day 3. Transform your Circuit

How do I discover my circuit? Use the Stop a Trigger Cycle

To find your circuit, follow the instructions below. If you are using EBT technology, start at the Check In icon, and select Brain State 4 and the Stop a Trigger option. Move through the lead-ins to discover your circuit. Keep your sense of humor! The reptile would be happy to keep you from expressing A+ Anger until your mind goes blank. Below is step-by-step guidance for discovering your first wire.

Discover the Circuit!
Use the Stop a Trigger Lead-Ins

- The situation is . . .
- What I'm most stressed about is . . .
- I feel angry that . . .
- I can't stand it that . . .
- I hate it that . . .
- I feel sad that . . .
- I feel afraid that . . .
- I feel guilty that . . .
- OF COURSE I would do that, because my unreasonable expectation is . . .

---

1) Say What is Bothering You
The situation is . . . What I'm most stressed about is . . .

In describing the situation, complain about your overeating – This accomplishes two things: 1) It ramps up stress, because only when we are in stress can we unlock the circuit so we can change it, and 2) it describes the situation so we can focus on the Food Circuit and activate it. Be sure to complain about your overeating. State the one thing that bothers you the most!

Do not state any feeling words, such as saying that you hate it that you overeat. Using words to state feelings reduces stress, and in this tool, we want to increase stress. That's how we can activate the wire related to our overeating that is stored in the lowest possible drawer of the brain. The lower in the brain the wire, the more strongly it drives excesses, so the more important it is to rewire. Just complain. Complain mightily! State the facts.

EXAMPLE: *The situation is . . . I am completely out of control with food. This is ruining my joy. I don't know what to do about it. I think about food all the time. I tell myself I am going to stop, but by the evening, I'm eating everything in sight. What I'm most stressed about is . . . I am completely out of control of my eating.*

2) Unlock the Circuit
I feel angry that . . . I can't stand it that . . . I hate it that . . .

Roust out that wire with A+ Anger – Express anger about your overeating. Stay on the topic of overeating. Why do we express such strong anger? We're now at the 4th Drawer of the brain; however, the reptilian brain is still laughing at us. It knows we're not serious. It believes we're going to let it off the hook and it's going to hold onto that circuit, perhaps for the rest of our lives. We may not have a food wire in the 5th Drawer of the brain, but if we do, nabbing and rewiring it will have the most impact.

To unlock that circuit, we need to be furious! So, we downshift into fury, name-calling, shaming, and blaming. We fight fire with fire. Expletives? Perfect! They are a sure sign that we are in that 5th Drawer and grabbing hold of that fight-or-flight drive to overeat that is encoded in the Food Circuit.

 Watch for the unlocking moment!

The sign that you have expressed strong enough anger to roust out and unlock that circuit? The brain turns off for a second or two. We're oddly quiet. This is the unlocking moment, the sign every EBT participant watches for. It is a sign that we are doing the deeper work, rewiring the circuits of hurt, trauma, addiction, compulsion – and that we are healing! Once our mind shuts off, then we pause. We take three deep breaths to connect with our bodies and move from expressing feelings to feeling feelings, slowing it way down. This is important! Feeling feelings takes time. Soon sadness begins to flow.

EXAMPLE: *I feel angry that . . . I can't stop overeating. I can't stand it that . . . food controls my life. I HATE it that . . . How dare you control me! I am furious! How %$#@!!! What an old, rusty, gnarly, stupid wire. I hate that I have this wire. I hate that I stuff myself with food. I HATE IT, I HATE IT . . . I HATE IT!!!* (The mind turns off for a moment and then sadness flows. The circuit is now unlocked!)

3) Discover the Hidden Message
I feel sad that . . . I feel afraid that . . . I feel guilty that . . .
OF COURSE I did that, because my unreasonable expectation is . . .

State one feeling, then pause and feel It – You've cracked open that circuit and now it's time to release the pressure of its emotional contents. Long ago, the stress of the moment was stuffed into that circuit, and ever since it has been rumbling around inside you. No more! The trick is to switch gears from expressing emotions at Brain State 4 or 5 to connecting with your body at Brain State 3. In that state you can feel your feelings and release that stress. You can feel your feelings and learn from them. *Do this for each of the three feelings, following the order of the lead-ins.*

For each feeling, you state the lead-in. Start with "I feel sad that . . ." and pause. Wait for words to bubble up into your conscious mind to complete the sentence. Stay on the topic, which is your complaint about food. Feel the sadness until it fades, about 10 to 20 seconds. Do not talk. Just feel your feeling until it fades. Then go on to the next lead-in, which is "I feel afraid that . . ." and do the same.

Then go on to "I feel guilty that . . ." The guilt is very important. This is not about shame, but about what you believe you could have done differently, what your part in the situation is. By finding your part in it, your hunter-gatherer brain will direct you right to the wire that is the problem. That wire made it perfectly reasonable for you to do that! We obey our unconscious, primitive circuits as a survival strategy. The problem is not you, it's that old wire!

EXAMPLE: (After taking several deep breaths to ease stress and access the deepest feelings possible) *"I feel sad that . . . I am out of control with my eating . . . I feel afraid that . . . I will always be out of control with my eating . . . I feel guilty that . . . I keep overeating even though I tell myself I will stop."*

Once you have identified your part in it (guilt), nurture yourself. A Stress Circuit made you do that! With an understanding and loving voice, say, "OF COURSE I did that, because my unreasonable expectation is . . ." and wait for words to bubble up. Once they appear in your mind, do not analyze the words. Trust them. Do not question the meaning of these words. This is not a logical process. The test of whether these words "match" the wordless message stored in your unconscious mind is if you have a "body feel" that they ring true. If the words do not ring true, circle back to the I feel guilty lead-in and repeat the process until they do. When the words match the emotional circuit's message, you will have nailed your cycle. When you state the words, your body will relax, and you will feel a slight glow. You may even be at Brain State 1, experiencing a surge of dopamine from finding your circuit.

Use the structure: I get my _____ from _____. These Stress Circuits are false associations between a fight-or-flight drive to meet a need and whatever we did to try to meet that need during some random experience in our life. That moment changed us. Before then, food was just food, but the circuit encoded a fight-or-flight drive to overeat. Rather than being at peace with food, that distorted, intense drive made it virtually impossible NOT to overeat!

Part of the fun of hunting down unwanted circuits and crushing them is to find a "pure gold" wire. That's a wire that is stored very low in the brain, usually in the 5th Drawer. This wire drives your most extreme eating style, the one that makes you feel as if you are completely out of control. Or, it might give you the illusion you are in complete control for the first time. Either way, it is strong, and by rewiring it, legions of other weaker circuits are cleared away, too.

These pure gold circuits are "survival circuits" as they are extreme, and they are stored in the 5th Drawer. Although you can use a generic message of **I get my safety from food**, there are other words that may ring true for you in the 5th Drawer, such as, I get my existence from overeating or I get my survival from eating sweets.

Experiment until the words ring true – To find an unreasonable expectation that rings true, you might need to do several Cycles or keep repeating the lead-ins "I feel guilty that . . ." and "OF COURSE I did that, because my unreasonable expectation is . . ." and digging deeper into your brain. Stick with it until one rings true. When it rings true, the message in the emotional wire and the words from the neocortical mind match! Now you have a conscious representation of the unconscious mind. You can use that statement to fry and transform the circuit.

EXAMPLE: *"OF COURSE I would do that, because my unreasonable expectation is . . . I can get the love I did not get during my childhood from eating a lot of food . . . no, that's not quite right . . . I think I'm listening to my thinking brain. I'll do it again. OF COURSE I would do that, because my unreasonable expectation is . . . I get my love from . . . food. That's better, but it still doesn't ring true. OF COURSE I would do that, because my unreasonable expectation is . . . I get my safety from . . . overeating. That feels right. That's my circuit. I crave safety. That rings true."*

 The words must ring true!

For the rest of the day, feel your feelings, and be aware of your circuit. Seeing that circuit just as it is – an extraneous wire that a random life event encoded in your brain – is often quite an emotional experience. For the first 30 minutes after you do your Cycle, the synaptic connections in the wire are very fluid, and by being aware of that wire, you can have the most impact on changing it. Between 30 minutes and two hours after discovery, the synapses are still open, so focusing your attention on the emotions that were generated by the circuit is particularly helpful.

Six hours after your Cycle the rewiring window closes, and although you can still impact the circuit, the synapses between the neurons have solidified and the hippocampus has stored them in long-term memory – for now!

Do you have a 5 Circuit? These words may bubble up!		
Safety	Survival	Existence
Protection	Power	Security

We can reactivate them later, but the rewiring window has shut. This is why the first day of the three-day rewiring plan is so powerful!

I am a pediatric nurse and well-versed in nutrition. I have always attributed the weight gain I've had in the last 10 years to my overindulgence in sweets. The problem was my bad habits and lack of willpower. When I did this Cycle, the words that appeared in my mind were: I get my existence from stuffing myself with sweets. I thought, "Where did that come from?" It didn't make sense to me until about four hours into my rewiring window when I realized that my mother had the same wire. That circuit was probably encoded in my unconscious memory system before the age of three. Astonishing!

Travel back on your circuit. As you become more comfortable with executing these "Discovery Cycles," you will learn how to reliably activate A+ Anger. That strong emotion unlocks very old circuits and circuits encoded during high-stress times and delivers an unlocking moment. Your EBT work will deepen. Sometimes, right after doing a Cycle that includes an unlocking moment, your mind will "travel back" on that circuit. Think of it as a trip through the past to a moment when the circuit was encoded or strengthened. This Travel Back is only possible when you happen to reach a very deep circuit, but you can always give it a try! Just focus on the place in your body where you feel stress, then say to yourself, "I have felt that sensation before!" Turn your attention to wondering about the past and notice any images that arise. If an image arises, you might even see yourself in a situation in which you turned to food to meet a safety need. You needed safety from connecting with yourself and others, not from overeating. You can even imagine yourself stepping into the image and comforting your past self. This can be a very loving and powerful experience. You are wiring in reconnecting to yourself, rather than to food.

Ask questions about your circuit and do Cycles to grieve the losses. Six or more hours after your Discovery Cycle, when the rewiring window has closed, you might want to ask yourself questions, such as: Is it an intergenerational circuit? Did a parent or someone else close to you have that circuit? If you have a sense of when it was encoded, what changes, losses, or upsets occurred within one year of that time? Help fill in the pieces of the puzzle about your story.

What if this discovery day stops being fun? If you do not find this to be fascinating, exciting, or illuminating, chances are that you are stressed. Do five Cycles to clear the stress. Cycle about anything, such as, the experience that encoded the wire, the fact that you did not know it was there, or the reality that the circuit has been harmful to you. Some people are stressed about giving up food. No worry there! We NEVER give up overeating! When the wire has been transformed, the drive to overeat vanishes. We eat healthy because our natural healthy eating style kicks in!

Each Cycle counts. If you need help with a circuit, get peer support (family member, friend, or connection buddy) or coaching from an EBT provider. Each Cycle clears away the past, so you have more peace and power from within.

Use the checklist on the next page to guide your way in discovering your Food Circuit.

The words of the unreasonable expectation of circuits generally follow the formula "I get my (need) from (food) ."

Discover Your Food Circuit
I get my _____ (need) _____ from _____ (food) _____.

There are two columns at the bottom of the checklist.

The "*I get my . . .*" checklist includes the five basic needs that the brain seeks: safety, love, comfort, pleasure, and purpose. This list includes additional words that may more accurately convey safety needs: survival, existence, protection, security, power, and nurturing.

The ". . . *from feeling*" checklist includes words related to stress eating, that is, how the wire tells you to use food in order to meet that need.

Discover the hidden message in that wire so that you can rewire it!

This is your first circuit. Be gentle with yourself. You do not have to do this perfectly. Once you learn this skill, you will have it for life! Before using the Rewiring Checklist, see page 277 for a list of ways to enhance your EBT experience. Join the EBT community, print out the companion forms for this book, or if you have questions, call in and chat with me. Congratulations on launching the discovery of your Food Circuit!

The Rewiring Checklist
Day 1. Discover Your Food Circuit

Say What is Bothering You:

- The situation is . . . (Complain about overeating.)
- What I'm most stressed about is . . . (Say what bothers you the most about overeating.)

Unlock the Circuit

- I feel angry that . . .
- I can't stand it that . . .
- I hate it that . . .

Discover the Hidden Message

- I feel sad that . . .
- I feel afraid that . . .
- I feel guilty that . . .
- OF COURSE I would do that, because my unreasonable expectation is . . .

I get my:	from:	
☐ Safety	☐ Food	☐ Eating rapidly
☐ Love	☐ Carbs	☐ Smelling food
☐ Comfort	☐ Sugar	☐ Chewing food
☐ Pleasure	☐ Eating sweets	☐ Swallowing food
☐ Purpose	☐ The taste of food	☐ Nibbling on food
☐ Survival	☐ Overeating	☐ Denying myself food
☐ Existence	☐ Stuffing myself	☐ Dieting
☐ Protection	☐ Binge eating	☐ Restraining myself
☐ Security	☐ Feeling too full	☐ Purging
☐ Power	☐ Getting a sugar high	☐ Obsessing about food
☐ Nurturing	☐ Eating large amounts	☐ Having a food problem
☐ Other _____	☐ Stuffing/starving	☐ Other _____

Success Check Day 9

- **Daily Success**

☐ I continued my Joy Practice with 10 Check Ins and 10 Joy Points.

☐ I discovered my Food Circuit.

☐ I made one or more community connections for support with discovering my circuit.

- **Did I pass the Success Check?   YES   NO**

If you did not, stay with this activity for one more day, then move on.

- **My Amazing Learning:**

_____

- **My Biggest Accomplishment:**

_____

- **My Biggest Challenge:**

_____

Congratulations!

You have completed Day 9 of The Joy Challenge.
Your next step is Day 10. Negate Your Food Circuit.

Day 10. Negate Your Food Circuit

You've discovered your Food Circuit! Now it is time to move to the second step of the EBT 3-Day Rewiring Plan. Let's negate it.

We're going to confront that unreasonable expectation with a strong statement that we can NOT get our safety, love, comfort, pleasure, or purpose from food, whether it's eating junk food, binge eating, or any unwanted way that we use food in our lives. That wire's message is ridiculous! As always, your job is to make this a ton of fun! We'll use Power Boosters to weaken that wire faster. Sounds fun, right?

Let's Weaken that Food Circuit
• **Do not ask yourself to stop overeating.** • **Instead, change the circuit that drives it.** • **As the circuit changes, your eating will change!**

Why

Before transforming the circuit into a message that sounds reasonable, we negate it. We need to take this intermediate step of weakening the old unreasonable expectation to follow the rules of neuroscience.

Neuroplasticity is based on Hebb's Law: *Neurons that fire together wire together and become stronger. Neurons that fire apart wire apart and become weaker.* Circuits only change through experience, and only the most emotionally-charged experiences are strongly remembered by the brain. The combination of discovering the circuit and repeatedly and intensively negating it with the opposite (mutually exclusive or orthogonal) message is just what we need.

Why is a very precise technique needed?

By stating the unreasonable expectation first, such as "I get my love from food," we activate the circuit and unlock it. Then, by negating the circuit, we tell the brain that it is not true. That weakens the circuit, readying it for transformation to a new, reasonable expectation on the last day of the three-day rewiring plan.

Fight-or-flight circuits do not change easily

The brain wants to hold onto these faulty circuits that deliver hidden ridiculous messages like food is going to make us feel loved or we have no way on Earth to get pleasure but by eating sugary foods that make us nauseated, bloated, and hungry! To change that wire, we need to use a Grind In with passion and lots of repetitions! Break down that circuit!

Touching those circuits activates a stress response

These circuits are stored in the brain with an eye to making it nearly impossible to change them unless we are at the same level of stress activation in which they were encoded. Even then, when we activate them, the reptilian brain is not happy. It believes that these circuits saved our lives, so once we target a circuit, we must be very careful to work with the reptile rather than needlessly stressing it. Too much stress and we go to a Brain State 5, a full-blown stress response, and our efforts to change the circuit shut down.

Weakening the circuit is an essential step

We take time to weaken the circuit because if we change the expectation too rapidly and without taking away some of its strength, the reptile will reject the message. To weaken the circuit, we must first stress-activate it, either saying the unreasonable expectation or by noticing that the circuit has been activated by daily stress. Once the circuit is activated, pause for one to 10 minutes until you are at Brain State 3. Perfect! The message you give the brain now will weaken that wire!

Is it true that you should NOT use the word NOT?

A commonly-discussed rule of changing circuits is to NOT use the word NOT in a corrective message. This rule applies when we are clearing out the top drawers of the brain. However, the circuits in the bottom drawers function differently. The unreasonable expectation must be confronted with the experience that it is not true. The negation accomplishes that and weakens the circuit. The brain can "hear" the word NOT because we state it very strongly, making it stand out like neon! The rest of the statement is very monotonal and the NOT is loud, emotional, vibrant, and strong so that the brain cannot miss it!

With those ideas in mind, let's look at what we actually do to weaken that Food Circuit and begin to break free of its hold over us.

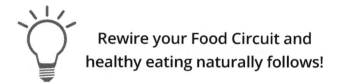

Rewire your Food Circuit and healthy eating naturally follows!

How

To negate your Food Circuit, first stress-activate it. For example, say, "I get safety from eating junk food." If you happen to be eating junk food, then notice that you get your safety from that. You'll be in stress, which is perfect. Then say, "I can NOT get safety from eating junk food." Again, state it very slowly at first, then ramp it up and ridicule the circuit. If you like, sing or dance or stomp when you are negating it. The more emotionally-charged the experience, the better the rewiring results.

2 Stages of Negating Your Food Circuit Example
SLOW: Repeat 3 to 6 times I . . . can . . . NOT . . . get . . . my love . . . from . . . eating sweets. RAMP UP: Repeat 3 to 6 times That does NOT give me the love I need. That's ridiculous! I can NOT get love from eating sweets. That's impossible!

SLOW – State it slowly the first three to six times

State the negated expectation very slowly. Don't scare the reptile. Say it so slowly that it almost hurts. The more slowly you state it, the deeper in the brain it will go. If you state it quickly at first, the brain stress will be so high that the prefrontal cortex cannot stay flexibly aware of your feelings. We disconnect from feeling our feelings in our body, and that connection is essential for self-directing our emotional plasticity. Start with stating the negation one word at a time. Pause between each word so that the reptile can let off steam.

RAMP UP – Ridicule that circuit three to six times

After stating the negation three to six times, you'll notice that your feelings start shutting down. The emotional vividness of the statement dulls. We need strong emotions in order to strengthen the new memory. Over the years, we have noticed that participants who were seeing better results actually made fun of their circuit. They used a ramped-up negation of the wire – saying, that's ridiculous! By making fun of the circuit, we "externalize" the wire, so we experience more power and pleasure while short-circuiting any latent shame that could arise.

Keep it fun – Sing or dance or scream it!

To lock in the incremental change in the wire, we need a burst of dopamine which we can get with this simple technique. As you negate the circuit, be sure to add a dose of dopamine in a way that works for you. Some people use an enthusiastic voice, others say it standing up, even while they are dancing. This celebration that you really cannot get your need met by that response is exhilarating.

I am committed to crushing my wire that tells me that I get my power from stuffing myself with food. First, I negated it for 30 minutes straight. I started slowly, but before long I was singing it, jumping around, and yelling it. I think I busted that circuit with the first 150 because I was so passionate. It was a celebration of my freedom from that stupid wire! Woo-hooo!

Tips on Negating Your Food Circuit
• You are not telling yourself to stop overeating.
• You are telling yourself that overeating does not work.
• Overeating does not meet the need you have.
• Even if you ate constantly, it would not meet your need.
• Do not force yourself to change your eating.
• Change the wire and changes in eating will follow.

Example (All Grind In Clusters count as 10 Grind Ins)

SLOW

* I . . . can . . . NOT . . . get . . . COMFORT . . . from . . . CARBS . . . (pause)
* I . . . can . . . NOT . . . get . . . COMFORT . . . from . . . CARBS . . . (pause)
* I . . . can . . . NOT . . . get . . . COMFORT . . . from . . . CARBS . . . (pause)
* I . . . can . . . NOT . . . get . . . COMFORT . . . from . . . CARBS . . . (pause)
* I . . . can . . . NOT . . . get . . . COMFORT . . . from . . . CARBS . . . (pause)

RAMP UP

* That's ridiculous! I can NOT get all my comfort from carbs.
* Self-medicating with carbs is not the answer.
* I can eat carbs all day and night but they will NOT give me the comfort I need!
* That's RIDICULOUS! I can NOT get comfort from eating carbs!
* Using carbs as my security blanket? Totally RIDICULOUS!
* I can't comfort myself by stuffing myself with carbs. HOW UTTERLY RIDICULOUS!!

How many times do you repeat your Grind In?

The goal is to weaken the circuit enough so that the reptilian brain will happily accept a new expectation. When the circuit is weakened, it's easier for the brain to override the message.

The stronger your Food Circuit, the longer you must pause in order to return to Brain State 3 and the more repetitions will be required. It takes as many repetitions as it takes, however, a general guideline is based on where that circuit is stored in the brain. If your Food Circuit is a weak one, meeting a need for pleasure or comfort, you may only need 50 repetitions. What if your Food Circuit is strong, say in the 4th or 5th Drawer? Then it will take a huge amount of repetitions and every bit of passion, enthusiasm, and power you can express through your words, vocal tone, and body will help! It's just a wire. You can weaken it!

How much negating do we need to do?

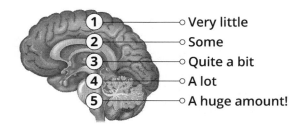

1 — Very little
2 — Some
3 — Quite a bit
4 — A lot
5 — A huge amount!

How do you keep it fun?

There is a very simple way. First, notice if it is not fun. When you aren't excited to zap that wire, do not do it! It will be a waste of your time to negate that wire until you have processed your emotions about it. That lack of enthusiasm is your brain's way of telling you that there are emotions to process prior to dismantling your circuit. Heed that message. Our saying "If it's not fun, it's not EBT" is based on neuroplasticity research. When the brain is "ready" to rewire a circuit, you may feel slightly scared, but a big part of you will say, "Let's have at it. I want to smash that wire!"

This is part of the process of rewiring emotional circuits. Again, when it is NOT fun, stop and do five Cycles. Then check to see if it sounds like fun to negate your circuit. If it doesn't, do another five Cycles. It takes as long as it takes. The reptile is watching us and fuming! Do as many Cycles as you need to do, then **negate that circuit with enthusiasm and joy!**

If it's not fun, then do 5 Cycles.
Grieve the loss, so that it's fun again.

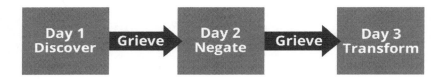

I stopped having fun negating the circuit, so I did Cycles to grieve. I was angry that I had to give up food. My unconscious mind was still telling me to diet. I do not have to stop overeating. That's ridiculous! I have to fry my food wire. After I fry it, my food drive will naturally fade. Negating the wire sounded like fun again!

Keep it Fun!
• Do not grieve and do Grind Ins at the same time.
• Do one or the other.
• If it's not fun to do Grind Ins, then do five Cycles.
• When it sounds like fun again, do Grind Ins.

To boost the rewiring power of your Grind In, try some of the techniques below whenever you think your Food Circuit might be activated. When you have a strong urge to eat when your body is not hungry, the synaptic connections of your Food Circuit have become fluid. The wire is hot or online and the connections between the neurons are open to change. If we "feed" that circuit a new message, the wire (memory) will be updated.

Power Boosters for your Food Circuit

- Use your Grind In when craving sweets.
- State it before, during, or after a meal.
- Grind it in when snacking or nibbling on food.
- State it when seeing or smelling food.
- Use your Grind In while binge eating.

This changes your relationship with food. Any food cue is a good thing! It is a momentary experience in which you could have remarkable success in weakening or breaking an old wire that was encoded through no fault of your own and has been telling you a big fat lie. By negating it when your Food Circuit is activated, you are changing your unconscious mind. You are inserting a new message that is truthful. Over time, the unconscious mind changes and so does your eating.

Have fun negating this wire! Be playful. You do not have to do this perfectly. Just charge forward and negate the old message. Your wire will begin to change!

The Rewiring Checklist
Day 2. Negate Your Food Circuit

I activated my Food Circuit by stating my unreasonable expectation, then paused until I was at Brain State 3. Then I negated it:

- **SLOW**
  I can NOT get my _____ from _____ .

- **RAMP UP**
  That's ridiculous! I can NOT get my _____ from _____ .

  I negated it: 50   75   100   125   150   200 _____ times.

I boosted the power of my Grind In (one or more ways):

- ☐ Using my Grind In when craving sweets
- ☐ Stating it before, during, or after a meal
- ☐ Grinding it in when snacking or nibbling on food
- ☐ Stating it when seeing or smelling food
- ☐ Using my Grind In while binge eating

Success Check Day 10

- **Daily Success**

☐ I continued my Joy Practice with 10 Check Ins and 10 Joy Points.

☐ I negated my Food Circuit.

☐ I made one or more community connections for support with negating my circuit.

- **Did I pass the Success Check?   YES   NO**

If you did not, stay with this activity for one more day, then move on.

- **My Amazing Learning:**

_____

- **My Biggest Accomplishment:**

_____

- **My Biggest Challenge:**

_____

Great Work!

**You have completed Day 10 of The Joy Challenge.
Your next step is Day 11. Transform Your Food Circuit.**

Day 11. Transform Your Food Circuit

Let's transform your Food Circuit. Today we will create a Power Grind In that not only dismantles that old wire but creates a new wire that activates surges of chemicals in the opposite direction.

The new circuit will awaken in you a desire to eat healthy, so that it is more fun to eat a crisp red apple when you're hungry than it is to consume sugary, artificial foods in the absence of body hunger.

To transform your Food Circuit, you will decide on a new message that tells you what to do, that is, to connect with yourself, to approach food in a new way, and to be aware of the reward that motivates you to eat in that way.

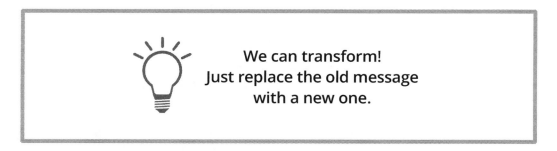

We can transform!
Just replace the old message
with a new one.

When we are running a stress eating wire, the circuit causes us to disconnect from ourselves, missing out on all the sensations and emotions that make us eat healthy intuitively.

We follow the wire's dictates, such as getting our safety from food, and our reward is artificial, such as the brief high of a sugar rush. The wire tells us to disconnect from ourselves, use an unhealthy approach to food, and to get by for the moment with an artificial reward.

A New Wire Replaces the Old One

	Connect	Food Approach	My Reward?
OLD WIRE I get my safety from . . .	disconnecting from myself	eating sweets	(artificial) a sugar high
NEW WIRE I get my safety from . . .	connecting to myself	eating healthy	(natural) vibrancy

The new instruction must have three components that counter the old wire, that is, to connect within, to use a more effective approach to food, and to feel a surge of reward that is natural.

To deliver that new instruction, we will use our prefrontal cortex and make a personal decision what message we want encoded in our unconscious mind. Then we will state that message to ourselves throughout the day or whenever that circuit begins to be activated.

Why

The purpose of the Power Grind In is to deactivate the Stress Circuit in real time, switching it to a Joy Circuit that reduces stress and activates a surge of neurotransmitters, which feels great! Basically, we give the brain a more effective response.

To accomplish this, the new statements need to directly confront the old statements on three counts. One is to check in or connect within rather than checking out or disconnecting. Without being checked in and connected, we have little or no power over the reptile!

Next, we add a new emotional approach, since the brain will continue its old response until we encode a new and better one. Last, we absolutely must install a natural reward (earned rewards of purpose are the best) which will deliver a dopamine spurt that makes using this new circuit sound like a great idea.

Once you've created this new statement, it's essential to learn to express it in an effective and handy way. The best method is to first remind the brain of your negation once, ridicule it with a hearty ramp up twice, and then grind in the new expectation three times.

Be sure to use a three-pronged statement (connect – approach – reward) so that you can punch the reptile in the nose and break this circuit!

The new instruction has three parts
• Connect – connect to yourself • Approach – use a new approach • Reward – savor your reward

How

Keep the message brief, clear, and sensitive to the reptile's strong urge to keep the circuit the way it is. Let's look more closely at how to construct your transformation statement for your Power Grind In:

Connect: Tell yourself to connect to your body, to the deepest part of yourself. You are instructing your prefrontal cortex (thinking brain) to turn its attention to your unconscious mind (emotional brain). It is that connection that makes us feel safe, loved, comforted, pleasured, and purposeful.

Approach: State what you're going to do when your Food Circuit has been activated. We'll look at a range of approaches, then do a brief visualization called an Imagine to finalize your plan. Develop a plan that will shut off that old wire and create a new one.

Reward: Which of the earned rewards will light up your brain with surges of powerful neurotransmitters so you joyfully unplug from overeating? Bring to mind your higher-order reward: Sanctuary, Authenticity, Vibrancy, Integrity, Intimacy, Spirituality, or Freedom.

Say how you will connect with yourself

Use a connect statement that is brief and clear to instruct your brain to connect within as your first defense against the activation of that Food Circuit.

Connect Statement Examples
• Connect with myself. • Check In. • Connect to the love inside me. • Connect to my body. • Take a deep breath. • Connect to the spiritual. • Honor my feelings. • Connect inside. • Be aware of my body. • Know my number.

What is your new approach to food?

The new approach is to be an effective parent to yourself. Imagine yourself about to overeat. What instruction do you need to hear? What follows are several approach statements. However, notice the words that bubble up from your unconscious mind. Go with those!

The Eat When Hungry Approach

One of the most effective ways to stop overeating is to make it a general policy that you do not eat unless you are hungry and you stop when you are just satisfied, not full. In 20 minutes, you will feel full. If your policy is to eat until you are full, you will feel stuffed and have a food hangover later on. That's not joy!

Eat When Hungry Approach Examples
• Do not eat unless I'm hungry.
• Eat when hungry and stop when hunger disappears.
• Eat only when I feel body hunger.

If you draw upon this concept, it's easy to say "no" to social overeating or pressure from family members to eat. You would no more eat when you are not hungry than go to the restroom when you do not have to relieve yourself. This approach is a way to have boundaries from the world, so that you control what you consume, rather than allowing the world or others to take away your power.

I am becoming more sensitive to my body. When I overeat, I feel sluggish. I used to eat right through that. I was numb. Not anymore! I eat when I am hungry and don't like the sluggish feeling after eating too much. I hate that. I follow my body's needs.

The Eat Healthy Foods Approach

Food can add stress to our bodies. Eating mainly Stress Foods can cause enough metabolic stress to make us sluggish or trigger a food hangover. Eating healthy reduces stress by keeping our blood sugar even, and avoiding those blood sugar lows. Also, if our food wire is really strong, then even small amounts of sugar or Stress Foods can trigger it. Some people adopt a "Zero Tolerance Policy" for eating a specific type of food (e.g., sugar). Why make life more difficult by playing with that wire?

Eat Healthy Foods Approach Examples
• Eat foods that make me vibrant.
• Eat foods that make me healthy and strong.
• Adopt a Zero Tolerance Policy.

My approach is to eat healthy. Sure, I eat Stress Foods sometimes, but not often. I think of the Joy Foods as natural medicine and prevention against anxiety attacks.

- Eat only when hungry.
- Eat mainly Joy Foods.
- Take a 12-hour food rest.

The EBT 3-Point Plan Approach

Another approach is to keep it very simple and follow the body's natural rhythms. Draw upon the wisdom of our evolutionary biology. Eat only if you are hungry and stop when the hunger disappears. Eat healthy foods but have enough Stress Foods to avoid feeling deprived. Have a food rest for 12 hours per day.

Awaken after resting from food for 12 hours. You'll be hungry. Food tastes great when we are hungry. Start eating when you are hungry and stop when you are just satisfied, not full. Eat a hearty breakfast and lunch. That's how our ancestors ate, which is why our stomach growls around midday. Have a light dinner, so that you sleep better, then have a food rest for 12 hours. Most people choose 7 p.m. to 7 a.m. for their food rest, but you can take it anytime. Why a food rest? This enables your body to burn up excess glucose and body starch (glycogen) and fat (triglycerides). Instead of the body holding onto extra weight, it's easier for the body to release it.

I like the body wise approach because I want to release weight. This gives me more flexibility to eat just what I need. I do not eat unless I am hungry and the food rest will probably help me sleep better.

EBT 3-Point Plan Examples
- Eat when I'm hungry, eat healthy, take a food rest
- Hungry – Healthy – Food Rested
- The EBT 3-Point Plan

The Meet My Need Approach

The last approach is to wire into our brain the drive to meet the original need for safety, love, comfort, or pleasure. It's a simple approach because you bypass any plan for food and zero in on the underlying need.

That's revolutionary. I tell myself to meet my basic need. If my need is comfort, I'll comfort myself. If my need is safety, I'll connect to the safe place inside me.

You can structure your approach statement to focus on the need, however, if the wire is deeper in the brain, it's often helpful to say what you will not do, too.

My Food Circuit was encoded during a lonely time when I was eight years old and my parents were really unhappy. There was a lot of turmoil and I went to food for love. Then I put on weight and was teased at school for being heavy. My approach statement is: I get my love from people, not food. I accept that food was my solution at the time, but I want real love now, not the sweetness of carbs.

Meet My Need Approach Examples

- Meet my true need, rather than overeating.
- Get my safety from inside me, not from food.
- Get my love from people, not from food.
- Comfort myself in healthy ways, not by overeating.
- Feast on natural pleasures, not on processed foods.
- Bring to mind my reward for eating healthy.

Where is your circuit stored?

The precise words you will use for your approach statement depend upon the drawer in which your Food Circuit is stored. The lower the drawer, the stronger your approach statement must be. **For example, if your desire to eat comes on gradually and keeps you in the 3 range**, then it's probably in the 3rd Drawer and a gentle reminder to connect within and eat healthy for the reward of vibrancy may be enough to deactivate your Food Circuit. **If your circuit is in the 4th Drawer,** being more directive is key. **If it is in the 5th Drawer**, be outright commanding. The 5th Drawer houses our compulsion and addiction circuits. And your drive to use that eating style may be that powerful. If it is, be blunt with your approach statement. Tell your brain to stop it!

Where is my circuit stored?

Location	Need	Strength of Drive
The 1st Drawer	Purpose	Very Low
The 2nd Drawer	Pleasure	Low
The 3rd Drawer	Comfort	Moderate
The 4th Drawer	Love	Strong
The 5th Drawer	Safety	Overwhelming

Which reward matters most to you?

Finish off your transformation statement by choosing the reward that motivates you to short-circuit that food wire. All seven of the rewards are important, but when it comes to this specific circuit and your Power Grind In that zaps that wire, which is the one that is most powerful for you?

The 7 Rewards	
• Sanctuary	Peace and power from within
• Authenticity	Feeling whole and being genuine
• Vibrancy	Healthy with a zest for life
• Integrity	Doing the right thing
• Intimacy	Giving and receiving love
• Spirituality	The grace, beauty, and mystery of life
• Freedom	Common excesses fade

The Food Circuit Imagine

One of the most rewarding ways to construct your transformation statement is by using the brain's astonishing capacity to imagine. This visualization will give you insights into just the instructions your brain needs to short-circuit that Food Circuit. Give it a try! We use this Imagine activity extensively in Advanced EBT because it reaches into the unconscious memory systems and changes them.

Relax: Set whatever limits are necessary to create privacy for yourself. Settle into a comfortable spot and begin to relax. Focus your attention on your body and your breathing. Breathe in through your nose and out through your mouth or in any way that is comfortable to you. When you are ready, begin to imagine.

Imagine: See yourself awakening in the morning and reminding yourself that you are creating joy in your life. You are doing your best to connect to the deepest part of yourself as you move through your day.

Now see yourself being triggered by that Food Circuit. Take a few moments and be aware of where you are . . . who is around you . . . how your body feels . . . and the thoughts that appear in your mind.

See yourself appreciating that this is a moment of opportunity to say to yourself just the words you need to hear to crush that wire and encode a new and better one. Imagine words appearing in your mind, clear instructions to connect with yourself . . . what would those words be? Take a few deep breaths. . . and after telling yourself to reconnect with yourself, what words appear in your mind about eating? What approach would be just what you need in that moment?

Notice that if you stay focused on your body, imagining that scene, the words will bubble up into your mind. Finally, what would motivate you to use that approach? Would it be Sanctuary, Authenticity, Vibrancy, Integrity, Intimacy, Spirituality, or Freedom?

Please take all the time you need and when you feel complete, use the upcoming checklist to record the transformation statement that feels right to you.

The Power Grind In (Counts as 10 Grind Ins)	
1 SLOW	Negate the expectation once.
2 RAMP UP	*Make fun of it twice. It's ridiculous!*
3 JOY	State your new expectation three times.

The Power Grind In

This Power Grind In is a tool that enables you to break free of this wire. You use it in daily life, beginning each time by stress-activating the circuit, either by stating the unreasonable expectation or when you come upon a "moment of opportunity" when daily stress activates it. Then you pause for a few moments or up to 10 minutes, until you are at Brain State 3. Then you negate the unreasonable expectation once, make fun of it twice, and finally repeat the transformation statement three times.

This Power Grind In comes in very handy as a cravings zapper tool in daily life. Use it preventively, during a stressful experience, and/or afterwards to further shift that old wire. Stressful moments speed up the process of breaking free from that old wire.

I just stuffed myself with way too much food, so the circuit has been activated by my daily life. I paused and appreciated that this wire is real. It's been in my brain since I was ten years old! I'm at Brain State 3. I'll use my Power Grind In. I can NOT get my love from feeling overly full . . . That's ridiculous! I can't get my love from feeling overly full. Food does not give me the love I need. Even if I ate until I was stuffed all day and all night, food could not give me the love I need. I get my love from connecting with myself, loving myself, and not stuffing myself with food. My reward: Sanctuary. I get my love from connecting with myself and giving myself so much love that I have no desire to stuff myself with food. My reward: Sanctuary. I get love from connecting with myself and loving myself so much that I have no desire to stuff myself with food. My reward: Sanctuary.

My unreasonable expectation is that I get my power from overeating. I can feel the stress in my body. I'm at Brain State 5. Okay, I'll pause for a few moments until I'm at Brain State 3. Okay, that took five minutes. That must be a deep circuit. Now I'll use my Power Grind In. Food does not give me the power I need. That's ridiculous! Even if I overate all day and all night, food could not give me the power I need.

I get my power from connecting inside, living a bold life, and eating healthy. My reward: Vibrancy. I get power from connecting inside, living a bold life, and eating healthy. My reward: Vibrancy. I get MY power from connecting INSIDE, living a BOLD life, and eating HEALTHY. My reward: Vibrancy!

The Power Grind In for Food: Example	
1 SLOW	I can NOT get my safety from food.
2 RAMP UP	*That's ridiculous!* I can NOT get my safety from food. *In fact, that's ridiculous.* My safety does NOT come from food. It feels like it, but it is NOT true.
3 JOY	I get my safety from connecting to myself, listening to my body, and eating healthy. My reward? Vibrancy. I get my safety from connecting to myself, listening to my body, and eating healthy. My reward? Vibrancy. I GET my safety from connecting to myself, *listening to my body, and eating healthy*. My reward? Vibrancy.

Use the checklist to record your Power Grind In for Food. Grind this in 100 or more times today. Want better results faster? Grind it in 200 times today. Each cluster counts as 10. Your brain will become comfortable with it. Then use this Power Grind In daily.

Watch for moments of opportunity to use your Power Grind In

It's easy to state the unreasonable expectation to give yourself that needed stress-activation, so the wiring changes are more lasting. However, once you have created your new Power Grind In, be in joyful anticipation of a craving. When one appears, seize the moment. Use your Power Grind In. Do not try to memorize your Power Grind In. These circuits are activated so quickly and so strongly that you will forget the words. It's essential to write your Power Grind In on a piece of paper or on your phone. Also, write it on the record of "My Power Grind Ins" on the last page of this book. Have your Power Grind In with you at all times. Who knows when the lizard brain could strike? In addition, use it four times daily, particularly during high-stress times.

This is your first Power Grind In. Use it with gusto! Congratulations on completing your first 3-Day Rewiring Plan!

The Rewiring Checklist
Day 3. Transform Your Food Circuit

After activating my Food Circuit by stating my unreasonable expectation, I paused until I was at Brain State 3. Then I transformed it:

- **SLOW**

  I can NOT get my _____ from _____.

- **RAMP UP**

  That's ridiculous! I can NOT get my _____ from _____.

- **JOY**

I get my: _____ from:

CONNECT	APPROACH	REWARD
☐ Connecting with myself	☐ Eating only when I am hungry	☐ Sanctuary
☐ Checking in	☐ Eating mainly Joy Foods	☐ Authenticity
☐ Connecting to my body	☐ STOP binge eating!	☐ Vibrancy
☐ Taking a deep breath	☐ Using the EBT 3-Point Plan	☐ Integrity
☐ Staying connected	☐ Eating for a higher purpose	☐ Intimacy
☐ Honoring my feelings	☐ Feasting on natural pleasure	☐ Spirituality
☐ Connecting inside	☐ Choosing healthy comforts	☐ Freedom
☐ Being aware of my body	☐ NOT seeking LOVE from food!	
☐ Knowing my number	☐ Creating safety from within	
☐ The deepest part of me	☐ Hungry – Healthy – Food Rested	
☐ Being present	☐ Having a Zero Tolerance Policy (food/eating habit)	
☐ Other _____	☐ Other _____	

I transformed it: 50   75   100   125   150   200 _____ times.

Success Check Day 11

- **Daily Success**

☐ I continued my Joy Practice with 10 Check Ins and 10 Joy Points.

☐ I transformed my Food Circuit and created my Power Grind In.

☐ I made one or more community connections for support with transforming my circuit.

- **Did I pass the Success Check?   YES   NO**

If you did not, stay with this activity for one more day, then move on.

- **My Amazing Learning:**

_____

- **My Biggest Accomplishment:**

_____

- **My Biggest Challenge:**

_____

Great Work!

You have completed Day 11 of The Joy Challenge.
Your next step is Day 12. Lifestyle Reset #2
Joy Breakfast and Sanctuary Time.

Day 12. Lifestyle Reset #2
Joy Breakfast and Sanctuary Time

As you settle into using your Power Grind In for Food, notice that you are more present, aware, and connected. Your interest might turn to lifestyle, upgrading how well it boosts your capacity to be at One.

Today we'll add two small but important resets of the brain for natural pleasures. One reset is the Joy Breakfast and the second is solo time devoted to the deeper work of EBT – Sanctuary Time.

Why

Not surprisingly, nutrition has a huge impact on both stress and neuroplasticity. Eating healthy not only reduces the physiologic stress caused by those blood sugar lows triggered by eating too much sugar, but has been associated with improved long-term memory (increased plasticity of neurons). What's more, excessive intake of sugary, processed foods can encourage hijacking of the brain's reward center to favor artificial pleasures.

All in all, with our goal of raising the brain's set point, and apart from rewiring our stress eating style, shifting toward eating healthy makes perfect sense.

The Power of Eating Healthy
• **Reduces brain stress**
• **Improves memory (neuroplasticity)**
• **Trains the reward center to favor healthy pleasures**

To make it easier to eat healthy without feeling deprived, start making more connections. The oxytocin surge from emotional connection is a powerful appetite suppressant. Just the way you may say, "How many Joy Points do I need to decrease my drive to overeat?", check to see how much loving connection you need to do the same! If it takes three five-minute connections to stop a binge, that's great. You can do three of them! There is no food hangover, but instead a deeper loving bond, which is a great investment in your health and happiness.

In EBT, we separate food into two categories: Joy and Stress. Joy Foods are whole foods and Stress Foods are processed foods. Think of foods based on evolutionary biology. Joy Foods include hunter-gatherer foods (fiber foods, healthy fats, and lean proteins). We emphasize including all three of these groups in a meal as that combination of foods is likely to keep hunger at bay for four to six hours. The protein-healthy fat combination has staying power for glycemic control and increases Peptide YY ("PYY"), the chemical in the intestines that signals us to stop eating. When PYY is high, we have absolutely no interest in food! There are also agrarian foods (other whole foods) if you prefer a plant-based diet.

The other food category is Stress Foods. These foods increase brain stress. They are lower in nutrient density (nutrition per calorie), can cause dopamine highs and lows that promote addiction, and can cause metabolic stress (the stress from blood sugar lows). Belly fat is often caused by the toxic combination of psychological stress and the metabolic stress amplified by processed foods.

We launch the healthy eating part of EBT with breakfast because breakfast sets the stress tone of the day. The stress hormone cortisol is high in the morning, to help us awaken, and the combination of high cortisol and consumption of Stress Foods can cause self-created hunger and the related ups and downs of our brain function and energy.

Check out some of the suggested breakfasts and give them a try. Consider food a form of natural medicine. Put into your body foods that add to your vibrancy – feeling healthy with a zest for life! Notice that the menu options listed are mainly Joy Foods but if you need small amounts of Stress Foods to avoid feeling deprived, then have them without a trace of guilt. Life is to be enjoyed!

Why PYY matters!

High protein meals increase PYY (Peptide YY),
the "stop eating" chemical, and as a bonus,
increase dopamine to enhance feelings of reward.

"I eat high protein meals to eat less naturally!"

How

The most important aspect of eating is that you eat only when hungry and stop when satisfied. That way you can feel full while avoiding that stuffed feeling. Always get to One (or as close as possible) before eating, as stress derails signals of satisfaction and hunger. See the Satisfaction Scale below. Also, eat mainly Joy Foods, but if you want Stress Foods, have them without guilt. Never deprive yourself! For breakfast, check off several breakfast ideas on the list below and try them. Also, you can create your own breakfast menu based on selecting mainly Joy Foods from the EBT Food List that appears later in this chapter.

The Satisfaction Scale

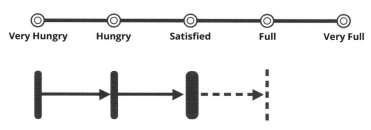

Get to One.
If you feel hungry or very hungry, then eat.
When you feel satisfied, stop eating. Wait 20 minutes.
You will feel full, without being overly full.

This Satisfaction Scale is really important because our needs for food are chemically driven. They change all the time. Sometimes you'll feel completely satisfied with very little food. Other times you'll need more. Listen to your body.

Also, as your set point moves up, your chronic stress will decrease. Chronic stress manufactures a drive to overeat. Also, as you use Joy Foods more and Stress Foods less, your insulin levels will go down and you will feel completely satisfied with less food. Last, as you score more Joy Points, you feel rewarded naturally without relying on food to boost your neurotransmitters.

Gradually, you will experience more freedom in your life. Food is still great, but you only yearn for it when you have body hunger. These adjustments in your food and appetite take time. Enjoy the journey!

Joy Breakfast Ideas

☐ **Eggs and Fruit**
2 eggs and 2 egg whites cooked in healthy fat, ½ grapefruit with cinnamon.

☐ **Avocado Eggs**
2 scrambled eggs cooked in healthy fat, topped with avocado and salsa.

☐ **Sausage Breakfast**
2 chicken or low-fat sausages and 1 egg cooked in healthy fat, 1 sliced orange.

☐ **Protein, Spinach, and Onions**
4 oz. salmon, chicken, or sardines sautéed in healthy fat with sliced onions and fresh spinach.

☐ **Eggs and Toast**
2 eggs cooked in healthy fat, 1 slice high-protein whole grain bread with healthy fat.

☐ **Eggs and Stuffed Celery or Apple**
2 eggs and 2 egg whites cooked in healthy fat, served with apple slices or a celery stick with pecan or almond butter.

☐ **Green Smoothie**
Blend 1 handful spinach, 1 c. almond milk, 1 banana, pear, apple, or orange with 1 scoop protein powder.

☐ **Power Smoothie**
Blend 1 scoop protein powder, 1 banana, 2 T. almond butter, 1 T. ground flaxseed, 1 c. frozen blueberries, and water to cover.

☐ **Strawberry Banana Smoothie**
Blend 1 scoop protein powder, 1 banana, and 1 c. strawberries plus almond milk to cover. Serve with a handful of pecans.

☐ **Eggs, Chorizo, and Berries**
2 scrambled eggs cooked with a few slices of chorizo sausage and fresh basil. Serve with fresh berries.

☐ **Sausage Patty Breakfast**
2 low-fat sausage patties and 1 sliced green apple sautéed in healthy fat. Sprinkle apple slices with cinnamon as they cook.

☐ Breakfast Bowl
1 c. berries sprinkled with 2 T. nuts, with 1 c. almond milk with 1 scoop protein powder.

☐ Leftover Protein and Fresh Tomatoes
Chicken or other lean protein reheated in healthy fat then tossed with sliced tomatoes and fresh basil.

☐ Salad Breakfast
A large plate of fresh greens with reheated lean protein (fish, poultry, or meat) and topped with olive oil and balsamic vinaigrette.

☐ Hawaiian Special
2 eggs and 2 egg whites cooked in healthy oil, served with 1 sliced papaya topped with a squeeze of lime.

☐ Chia Seed Smoothie*
Blend ½ c. cashews, 1 T. chia seeds, ½ t. vanilla extract, 1 c. ice cubes, and 1 banana with water to cover.

☐ Beet and Raspberry Smoothie*
Blend ¾ c. cooked beets, ¾ c. frozen raspberries, 1 c. almond milk, and 1 T. ground flaxseed with water to cover. Top with slivered almonds.

☐ Wheat Germ Smoothie
Blend ¾ c. Greek yogurt, ½ c. almond milk, 1 c. frozen blueberries, 1 T. wheat germ, and a few ice cubes with water to cover.

☐ Whole Grain Toast and Nut Butter*
Toast any whole grain bread that you like and top with any nut butter that appeals to you.

☐ Vegan Salad Breakfast*
A large plate of fresh greens tossed with ¼ c. nuts and ½ avocado cubed and topped with olive oil and balsamic vinaigrette.

☐ Quick Cottage Breakfast
¾ c. cottage cheese with ½ banana sliced and 1 T. toasted wheat germ.

☐ Yogurt and Fruit Breakfast
1 c. Greek yogurt with ½ c. fruit of your choice and 2 T. nuts of your choice.

* not a high-protein breakfast but rich in agrarian foods with high nutrient density

The EBT Food List
Joy Foods

Hunter-Gatherer Foods
These foods are rich in nutrient density (nutrition per calorie) and can decrease hunger, boost energy, and promote vibrancy.

1. The Fiber Group

Vegetables
- Acorn squash
- Artichokes
- Arugula
- Asparagus
- Bamboo shoots
- Banana squash
- Bean sprouts
- Beets
- Bok choy
- Broccoli
- Brussels sprouts
- Butternut squash
- Cabbage
- Carrots
- Cauliflower
- Celery
- Chard
- Chayote

- Corn
- Cucumbers
- Eggplant
- Endive
- Fennel
- Green onions/scallions
- Green peas
- Hubbard squash
- Jicama
- Kale
- Leeks
- Mushrooms
- Mustard greens
- Okra
- Onions
- Parsnips
- Pea pods
- Peppers
- Potatoes

- Pumpkin
- Radishes
- Romaine
- Scallions
- Shallots
- Snap peas
- Snow peas
- Spaghetti squash
- Spinach
- Sprouts
- Summer squash
- Sweet potato
- Swiss chard
- Tomatoes
- Water chestnuts
- Yams
- Yellow summer squash
- Zucchini

Fruits
- Apples
- Apricots
- Bananas
- Blackberries
- Blueberries
- Cantaloupe
- Cranberries
- Cherries
- Grapefruit
- Grapes
- Guavas
- Figs
- Honeydew melon
- Kiwis
- Lemons
- Limes
- Mangoes

- Melons
- Nectarines
- Oranges
- Papayas
- Peaches
- Pears
- Persimmons
- Pineapples
- Pomegranates
- Plums
- Prunes
- Raisins
- Raspberries
- Strawberries
- Tangelos
- Tangerines
- Watermelon

2. Healthy Fats

- Avocados
- Olives
- Omega 3 eggs
- Salmon
- Sardines

Nuts
- Almonds
- Hazelnuts
- Macadamias
- Peanuts
- Pecans
- Pistachios
- Walnuts
- Butters from the above

Seeds
- Flaxseeds
- Pumpkin seeds
- Sesame seeds
- Butters from the above

Oil
- Almond
- Avocado
- Canola
- Flaxseed*
- Hazelnut
- Macadamia

- Olive, extra virgin*
- Peanut
- Pecan
- Walnut

Salad Dressings
- Dressings made with vinegar or lemon and healthy oils

3. The Protein Group

Fish & Shellfish
- Barramundi
- Calamari
- Clams
- Cod
- Crab
- Halibut
- Haddock
- Herring, Atlantic
- Mackerel, Atlantic
- Mahi-mahi
- Mussels
- Ono

- Oysters, farmed
- Prawns
- Red snapper
- Salmon, Alaskan, wild
- Sardines
- Scallops, farmed
- Shrimp
- Sole
- Squid
- Tilapia
- Trout
- Tuna, albacore
- Tuna, yellowfin

Poultry & Meat
- Beef round steak
- Beef round, ground
- Beef flank steak
- Beef sirloin tip roast
- Buffalo
- Canadian bacon
- Chicken, ground
- Chicken breast
- Chicken drumsticks, skinless
- Chicken thighs, skinless
- Goat meat
- Ham, all fat removed

- Lamb steaks
- Pork chops, lean
- Pork tenderloin
- Sausage links, low-fat
- Sheep meat
- Turkey, ground
- Turkey breast
- Veal lean
- Venison

More
- Eggs
- Egg substitute
- Egg whites
- Protein powder

Agrarian Foods
These food are whole foods that provide important nutrients. For some people, these foods increase stress, hunger, and inflammation.

Grains
- 100% whole grain bread
- 100% whole grain cereals
- 100% whole grains cooked

Beans
- Legumes
- Beans

Milk Products
- Milk
- Yogurt
- Cheese

Stress Foods

Post Industrial Revolution Foods
The post-industrial revolution foods cause even more stress, hunger, and inflammation in humans.

Everything else!

Questions? Speak with a registered dietitian, physician, or nurse practitioner about the amounts of agrarian and industrial foods that are appropriate for you given your health status and risk factors for obesity, diabetes, heart disease, cancer, depression, anxiety, addiction, and other conditions.

In the Fiber Group, choose vegetables and fruits that are organic and farmed locally when possible. Rather than consuming juices, eat whole fruits and vegetables. In the Healthy Fats group, (*) these oils have exceptionally good healthy fat contents. In the Protein Group, emphasize consumption of fish and choose red meat in moderation, choosing natural, grass-fed meats cooked without frying or grilling when possible.

Be sure to enjoy your food. Again, eat slowly. Focus all your attention on the natural pleasure of eating food that delivers high-intensity well-being. Collect some Joy Points as you eat. Connect with yourself and eat slowly, savoring every bite:

- Notice the mouth-feel, taste, and pleasure in chewing and swallowing.
- Feel gratitude for your health to be able to eat.
- Be aware of your sensory pleasure in eating.
- Appreciate the joy of eating only when you are hungry.
- Feel grateful for your abundance, that you have access to food.
- Think about the people who contributed to your nourishment.

Appreciate yourself for taking a few moments to eat food that sustains your positive mood, high energy, and personal vibrancy throughout the morning and beyond.

Take Sanctuary Time for 10 Minutes

The tools of EBT can be used solo or with other people. The foundation for intimacy with others is intimacy with ourselves. That takes clearing away emotional clutter, doing lots of Cycles, and carving out from the busy schedule we might have to put being at ONE first, which requires solo time. Take 10 minutes per day to be alone and use the tools to clear away the day's stress. Find a quiet place and enjoy closing your eyes and relaxing as you use the tools. Establishing that pattern of taking 10 minutes daily, much like you would with a meditation practice, can have a grounding impact on your day. By setting limits and taking this time, there are many benefits to you and those around you.

Sanctuary Time
• A safe time to cycle through daily emotions • A way to honor the deeper work you are doing • Training the brain that emotional connection matters

My children are used to having constant access to me when I am home, and by telling them that they could not interrupt me for 10 minutes because I was having solo time, they perked up. Their mother has limits and cares about her inner life!

I schedule my Sanctuary Time when I come home from work. My habit had been to discuss the day with my partner, but most of my stories were complaints about people or projects. By taking those 10 minutes, I get myself to Brain State 1 or 2 and our entire conversation goes better. I like myself better when I'm at Brain State 1 or 2, rather than at Brain State 3 or 4.

You have completed the second lifestyle reset! Exercise, healthy eating and taking time for yourself will help strengthen your secure connection to the deepest part of yourself. Well done!

Success Check Day 12

- **Daily Success**

☐ I continued my Joy Practice with 10 Check Ins and 10 Joy Points.

☐ I reset my lifestyle in these three ways: Exercise, Joy Breakfast, and Sanctuary Time.

☐ I made one or more community connections for support with my lifestyle reset.

- **Did I pass the Success Check?   YES   NO**

If you did not, stay with this activity for one more day, then move on.

- **My Amazing Learning:**

_____

- **My Biggest Accomplishment:**

_____

- **My Biggest Challenge:**

_____

Congratulations!

**You have completed Day 12 of The Joy Challenge.
Your next step is Day 13. Discover Your Mood Circuit.**

Day 13. Discover Your Mood Circuit

You have created your first Power Grind In. Use it with gusto throughout the day and see if you can zap your Food Circuit right when it starts to arise. But bear in mind that emotional wires activate other emotional wires.

There are three "feeder circuits" that trigger the Food Circuit: Mood, Love, and Body. To stop stress eating, we also need to track those circuits down and transform them. We'll start with the Mood Circuit.

Mood Circuits are encoded when a fight-or-flight wire co-activates with a mood. Based on associative learning, the circuits couple, and strengthen our drive to trigger that mood even when small stresses come our way.

I am not that bothered by my Worry Circuit on its own, but if my stress level is really high and my Worry Circuit is fully triggered, I go rogue with food. I'll eat virtually anything I can get my hands on. I can't help it. My Worry Circuit triggers my Food Circuit.

The Mood Circuit

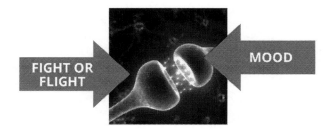

Three types of stressed emotions

Stressed moods are divided into three types: false highs, unnecessary lows, and numbness. They appear to be very different and, in their most extreme states, conventional psychology would label them as various disorders.

Using a neuroscience approach, they are just wires, and functionally, they share a characteristic: they keep us from being present to our balanced emotions that would point us to meeting our actual needs. When our Mood Circuit is activated, it causes us to abandon those helpful, healing feelings and escape into stuck, unbalanced emotions that lead nowhere good. Just the way food can be an escape from being present, so can moods.

Stressed Moods

Mood Type	Examples
False Highs	rebellious, all-powerful, manic, arrogant, frenzied, reckless, righteous, bullet-proof, chaotic, high
Unnecessary Lows	anxious, depressed, hostile, irritable, powerless, self-pitying, panicked, worried, discouraged, lost, ashamed, overwhelmed, disgusted, annoyed
Numbness	no feelings, shut down, numb, empty, detached, frozen, disconnected, zoned out, blanked out

The first type of stressed mood is a false high. We feel not just good, but so great that we miss out on the reality of the situation, as it is the grounding negative emotions (even a spark of them) that keep us sensible and responsive to real needs. We bite into a candy bar and it tastes so great that we have two of them. The consequences of our behavior elude us!

The second type of stressed mood is an unnecessary low. Lows are good for us if they are passing and alert us to a need, such as being hungry or lonely. However, these stressed emotions become stuck. If shame comes over us after a binge, we become absorbed in the shame rather than moving beyond the binge and taking a walk or accessing healthy pleasures.

The third type of stressed mood is numbness. We have no feelings. Often numbness is not the trigger to overeat, but the goal of overeating. When we focus on food and eating, we may "numb out" and the difficult emotions vanish.

These moods easily become persistent

It's normal to experience stressed emotions, and nobody is "present" to their feelings all the time. However, when a stressed mood is triggered often, the brain perceives it as a good thing. The mood, whether it is depression or hostility, frenzied or numb, is familiar, and we develop a really strong neural pathway in our brain for that mood, and trigger it repeatedly or chronically. It may feel bad, but the reptile within is exceedingly comfortable triggering it!

Why

Most of us have several Mood Circuits. We might have one that bothers us the most and others that dance in our heads at various times. In fact, it's normal to have one Mood Circuit that triggers overeating, another that encourages us to prolong our overeating episodes, and another one (the Mood Circuit dessert!) that follows stress eating episodes. We become familiar with these dancing moods and may even become more strongly attached to them than to the food!

The immediate goal of this book is to end overeating, so when you choose a Mood Circuit to rewire, consider selecting the mood that triggers your overeating. Put the other two "on the shelf" to rewire later, along with the mood that bothers you the most. Rewiring is a skill. By rewiring the Mood Circuit that triggers your Food Circuit, you will end overeating more rapidly. Also, with each rewire, your set point moves up and your skill in transforming circuits improves, too.

Mood Circuits Impact Overeating: Examples

Rewire Now: Before Eating	Rewire Later: While Eating	After Eating
Anxious	Numb	Ashamed
False High	False High	Numb
Depressed	Rebellious	Depressed

Anxiety definitely triggers me to eat, but I'm almost always anxious. When I'm on my way home from work, anxious, I start thinking about food, and then I have a craving. As soon as I arrive home, I overeat.

Depression triggers me to comfort myself with sweets, then I eat the sweets and go into a false high. When I'm stress eating, I feel normal, even good. It's the only time I feel that way. Afterwards, I beat myself up and feel ashamed. All three emotions are delicious in their own way. I'll rewire my feeder circuit of depression.

I come from a family of people who get their attention from feeling sorry for themselves. Some families have joy fests. Our family has pity parties. When my Pity Party Circuit is activated, I go right to food. I'm going to zap that one! Just because my family has pity parties, that doesn't mean that I have to.

How

To discover your Mood Circuit, bring to mind the mood that precedes your drive to overeat. Use the Stop a Trigger Cycle option in this book or, if you are using EBT technology, use the automated guides on your app and member home page. After one or more Cycles, your brain message (unreasonable expectation) that makes it perfectly reasonable that you'd experience that mood will bubble up in your mind. When the words that arrive in your mind ring true to you, that's your Mood Circuit!

Use this day to discover your Mood Circuit, sit with your feelings, visualize your circuit, and be aware of the words of that circuit. It was encoded without your permission or awareness. Being aware of your emotions during the six hours after you discover the wire is particularly helpful. This wire has been living within you for some time. You have a relationship with it!

Examples of Mood Circuits
• I get my safety from going numb.
• I get my comfort from worrying.
• I get my love from depression.
• I get my protection from feeling irritable.

Travel Back, Cycle, Journal, or Connect

If you want to explore the circuit some more, then either do a Travel Back or more Cycles. Perhaps explore whether or not it is an intergenerational wire. If you identified when this circuit was encoded, ask yourself what changes, losses, or upsets occurred within one year of the time.

If you like, create a "nickname" for your wiring. Why not keep it fun? Savor this time, as you are deepening your awareness of yourself and launching a new level of love, respect, and insight into who you are and where you have been.

Enjoy discovering your second Stress Circuit! Starting tomorrow, you'll begin dismantling it, so it will stop triggering your Food Circuit. The reward? More freedom and joy in your life!

The Rewiring Checklist
Day 1. Discover Your Mood Circuit

Say What Is Bothering You

- The situation is . . . (Complain about the mood that triggers you to overeat.)
- What I'm most stressed about is . . . (Say what bothers you the most about that mood.)

Unlock the Circuit

- I feel angry that . . .
- I can't stand it that . . .
- I hate it that . . .

Discover the Hidden Message

- I feel sad that . . .
- I feel afraid that . . .
- I feel guilty that . . .
- OF COURSE I would do that, because my unreasonable expectation is . . .

I get my:

- ☐ Safety
- ☐ Love
- ☐ Comfort
- ☐ Pleasure
- ☐ Purpose
- ☐ Survival
- ☐ Existence
- ☐ Protection
- ☐ Security
- ☐ Power
- ☐ Nurturing
- ☐ Other _____

from feeling:

- ☐ Anxious
- ☐ Depressed
- ☐ Hostile
- ☐ Irritable
- ☐ Powerless
- ☐ Self-pity
- ☐ Panicked
- ☐ Ashamed
- ☐ Abandoned
- ☐ Overwhelmed
- ☐ Worried
- ☐ Lost

- ☐ Rebellious
- ☐ All-powerful
- ☐ Manic
- ☐ Arrogant
- ☐ Righteous
- ☐ Bullet-proof
- ☐ No feelings
- ☐ Numb
- ☐ High
- ☐ Zoned out
- ☐ Disconnected
- ☐ Other _____

Success Check Day 13

- **Daily Success**

☐ I continued my Joy Practice with 10 Check Ins and 10 Joy Points.

☐ I discovered my Mood Circuit.

☐ I made one or more community connections for support with discovering my circuit.

- **Did I pass the Success Check?   YES   NO**

If you did not, stay with this activity for one more day, then move on.

- **My Amazing Learning:**

_____

- **My Biggest Accomplishment:**

_____

- **My Biggest Challenge:**

_____

Congratulations!

**You have completed Day 13 of The Joy Challenge.
Your next step is Day 14. Negate Your Mood Circuit.**

Day 14. Negate Your Mood Circuit

You've discovered your Mood Circuit, the one that triggers your stress eating style.

Even though the mood might not feel good, the brain has a "crossed wire," or mislearning, that this unhinged mood is going to give you safety, love, comfort, or pleasure.

We're going to weaken that circuit today so that it will be easier to start transforming it tomorrow.

Want to make it more fun, and therefore more effective? Use the new Power Boosters, including scented oils and nocturnal Grind Ins! Both are ways to deliver that new message to the brain in ways that start to update the wire and change it for the long-term.

**Clear away your Mood Circuit
to avoid triggering your Food Circuit.**

Why

We will negate that Mood Circuit because it is the next logical step toward rewiring it, and we need to rewire it! This neuroscience approach to stress eating is new to you. It's important to have success with stopping overeating, not only because that's the result you want from working your way through this book, but because once you see how powerful you can be by using these tools, you'll want to use them on other circuits, too.

To understand the importance of this Mood Circuit on your eating, imagine that the remnants of your Food Circuit are sitting at the bottom of your brain. That food wire is accustomed to being triggered by a mood and, as old circuits love to return to the limelight by being reactivated, it is patient. It will wait for the Mood Circuit to trigger it.

The utility of clearing the Mood Circuit is related to its nature. Mood Circuits can be triggered on many occasions. If we do not fry this circuit, in essence uncouple that false association between a basic need and that mood, the Food Circuit could have lots of opportunities to reappear.

Plus there is an added bonus in rewiring this circuit. The activations it triggers of other unwanted responses in daily life can be cleared away, too. All in all, rewiring this circuit is an excellent use of your time.

How

To negate your Mood Circuit, begin by activating it. For example, state, "I get safety from worrying." Pause for a few moments until you are at Brain State 3. This promotes lasting change in the circuit. Then say, "I can NOT get safety from worrying." State it very slowly at first, then ramp it up and ridicule the circuit. If you like, sing, dance, or stomp when you are negating it. The more emotionally-charged the experience, the better the rewiring results.

2 Stages of Negating a Mood Circuit	
SLOW	I . . . can . . . NOT . . . get . . . my . . . love . . . from . . . self-pity. I . . . can . . . NOT . . . get . . . my . . . love . . . from . . . self-pity. I . . . can . . . NOT . . . get . . . my . . . love . . . from . . . self-pity.
RAMP UP	That's ridiculous! I can NOT get love from pitying myself. Even if I pitied myself all day and night, it would NOT give me love. That's completely ridiculous! I can NOT get love from self-pity.

Example (All Grind In Clusters count as 10 Grind Ins)
SLOW
* I . . . can . . . NOT . . . get . . . SAFETY . . . from . . . being numb . . . (pause)
* I . . . can . . . NOT . . . get . . . SAFETY . . . from . . . being numb . . . (pause)
* I . . . can . . . NOT . . . get . . . SAFETY . . . from . . . numbing out . . . (pause)
* I . . . can . . . NOT . . . get . . . SAFETY . . . from . . . NUMBING . . . (pause)
* I . . . can . . . NOT . . . get . . . SAFETY . . . from . . . NUMBING OUT . . . (pause)

RAMP UP

- That's ridiculous! I can NOT get safety from numbing out.
- Numbing out does NOT give me safety.
- Unplugging from my feelings does NOT make me safe.
- That's ridiculous! I can NOT get safety from numbing out!
- How could numbness make me SAFE? Totally RIDICULOUS!
- Numbness is NOT my SAFETY BLANKET. No Way! How RIDICULOUS!!!

My Mood Circuit is definitely a 5 Circuit, as it is getting incensed. One moment I am calm, perhaps a little numb. Then something triggers my Hostility Circuit and I am so furious that it scares me. Instantly my Food Circuit goes off and I binge on carbs. I tricked that circuit! I used my hostility about being hostile to fire up my desire to crush this circuit. I negated it about 400 times and was singing, yelling, and screaming it (all in my head). I could hear myself yelling it, and my whole body was shimmering with emotion. It worked. That hostility circuit is nearly dead and gone. I'm ready to transform it.

My Mood Circuit is anxiety. It's a 3 Circuit, a comfort wire, as my mother gave me attention because I was anxious. I was the child that she worried about. Anxiety can NOT give me comfort now as an adult. It makes me seek comfort in food. Imagining that wire as a misconception in the brain, a mix-up between comfort and chronically feeling uneasy, helps me. I want freedom from that wire, so I stop overeating, but also because I want more joy in my life. I am going to negate that wire 100 or 1000 times until that mixed up association breaks. I want JOY.

Add Power Boosters to zap that Mood Circuit

Let's use some Power Boosters to weaken this Mood Circuit and create as much freedom as possible from that unbalanced emotional state. We are not in complete control of these wires. Some are simply stronger than others and require that we raise our set point to get relief. Also, the goal is not to be free of that mood. Brief periods of anxiety, depression, hostility, and more are part of breaking up old circuits and releasing our pent-up suppressed emotions. Rewiring the circuit keeps these emotions brief and productive!

Today's Power Boosters can speed your progress in weakening this circuit. Definitely live in joyful anticipation of the next activation of that circuit. You can exclaim, "Great news! I'm getting activated. That wire is unlocked and I can rewire that ridiculous message!"

Every day includes challenges, so when you start your day by saying, "I am creating joy in my life," add, something about your Mood Circuit, like, " . . . and zapping that Mood Circuit so it won't trigger me to eat sweets!" Anticipate a high-stress time when the wire is apt to be fired up, and grind in words that begin to weaken and crush it!

Power Boosters for your Mood Circuit

- Use your Grind In right when your circuit is triggered.
- Choose one challenging situation today and use your Grind In.
- State your Grind In before going to bed.
- Repeat your Grind In when you awaken in the night.
- Add essential oils with a scent to deepen your rewiring.

Also, take advantage of how easily the brain changes when we are asleep. The hippocampus consolidates the learning of the day into long-term memory when we are asleep. By doing Grind Ins right before going to sleep, or if you awaken during the night, you'll see better results. Some people drink water before retiring, to ensure they awaken in the night, so they can do Nocturnal Grind Ins.

Essential Oils Can Help!

Chamomile	Sandalwood	Lemon
Ginger	Rose	Bergamot
Lavender	Peppermint	Sage

The mechanism for improving neuroplasticity by using scents is based on the observation that scents go straight to the emotional brain. Creating an association between a scent and your Grind In is thought to intensify the experience of this new message and thus, promote more change in the circuit. If you want to try this, do Grinds Ins with a dab of scented oil under your nose or on your chest. Massage it into your skin or put a drop on your pillow at bedtime. The scent will continue to help grind in your message as you sleep.

This is your second time negating a circuit. Develop your own style for doing it, relying on repetition and strong emotions. It's a skill – a really important skill!

Let's transform that Mood Circuit. Let's do it!

The Rewiring Checklist
Day 2. Negate Your Mood Circuit

I activated my Mood Circuit by stating my unreasonable expectation, then paused until I was at Brain State 3. Then I negated it:

- **SLOW**

    I can NOT get my _____ from _____.

- **RAMP UP**

    That's ridiculous! I can NOT get my _____ from _____.

    I negated it: 50   75   100   125   150   200 _____ times.

I boosted the power of my Grind In (one or more ways):

☐   Using my Grind In right when my circuit is triggered

☐   Choosing one challenging situation and using my Grind In

☐   Stating my Grind In before going to bed

☐   Repeating my Grind In when I awaken in the night

☐   Adding essential oils with a scent to deepen my rewiring

Success Check Day 14

- **Daily Success**

☐ I continued my Joy Practice with 10 Check Ins and 10 Joy Points.

☐ I negated my Mood Circuit.

☐ I made one or more community connections for support with negating my circuit.

- **Did I pass the Success Check?   YES   NO**

If you did not, stay with this activity for one more day, then move on.

- **My Amazing Learning:**

_____

- **My Biggest Accomplishment:**

_____

- **My Biggest Challenge:**

_____

Congratulations!

You have completed Day 14 of The Joy Challenge.
Your next step is Day 15. Transform Your Mood Circuit.

Day 15. Transform Your Mood Circuit

You are about to create a Power Grind In to transform your Mood Circuit. Once you start thinking of a mood as an activation of a string of neurons, a "chain" in your brain, you can become practical about clearing it. The reptilian brain is not that smart and keeps reflexively sending you to that mood. That will not change unless you train your brain to change it. That's our task starting today.

Your Power Grind In is a personalized message that confronts the unreasonable expectation, then quite elegantly contradicts that message, thereby weakening it. Then it ridicules that unreasonable expectation. Finally, your Power Grind In replaces that old, ineffective message with a new, effective message of your choosing. It not only short circuits that "triggered" drive to adopt that mood, but using it repeatedly begins to rewire that circuit!

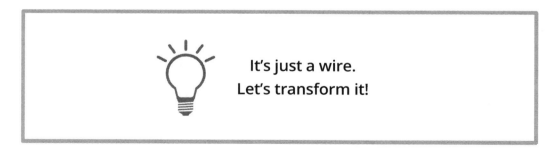

It's just a wire.
Let's transform it!

Why

The need to transform the circuit comes from the nature of the brain. The brain's two priorities (other than procreation) are survival and well-being. The Stress Circuits launch a survival drive that ends with a flourish of positive emotions. If survival-seeking is the main course of the meal, then a positive emotional surge is the dessert.

The challenge is posed by the fact that the old circuit, even one that is objectively unpleasant, such as my old Mood Circuit, which was: I get my nurturing from depression with a little self-pity thrown in, is perceived by the brain as safe and rewarding. It's safe because it is familiar and it's rewarding because it's familiar. You can see that the reptile likes to keep things the same!

So we must replace that old wire with a new one that feels safe. Repeating the new statement makes it more rewarding. So does having a clear instruction, as both the reptilian brain and the neocortex do not like ambiguity. Finding a reason for following through with the new instruction that is as delicious as the old one is essential. We use higher-order rewards because the brain's reward center lights up to them. Tell yourself that you are going to snap out of a grouchy mood because you should, and you will not get anywhere, but find a reason that matters to you, such as vibrancy, integrity, or freedom, and you're on your way to transformation.

How

The brain is very picky about your new statement. In fact, constructing it is a very intimate activity. It involves trying out various combinations of words that lay down a new and better brain pathway.

The structure of your transformation statement is dictated by needing to confront and overpower all three parts of the old circuit. By using a three-pronged Grind In, each part of the wire will be replaced.

If our Mood Circuit is deep in the brain, perhaps a 4 or 5 Circuit, that approach is particularly important. We're up against the inner lizard and need a Power Grind In that effectively punches that reptile in the nose!

Connect: Instruct yourself to turn your attention to your body and connect with yourself. Choose words that you want to hear, but be sure that your first step is to connect within. That curtails that activation of circuits that command you to unplug from yourself and plug into an unbalanced mood, such as anxiety, depression, hostility, or numbness.

Approach: State your new policy about processing emotions. All of us have thoughts and they are important, but it's effective emotional processing that is our ticket to pass through stress to joy. Plan your approach for doing that.

Reward: Which of the earned rewards will light up your brain with surges of powerful neurotransmitters so you joyfully unplug from that unwanted mood? Bring to mind your higher-order reward: *Sanctuary, Authenticity, Vibrancy, Integrity, Intimacy, Spirituality, or Freedom.*

Say how you will connect with yourself

It's easy to determine if the words you use to instruct yourself to connect will be effective. When you say them to yourself, you'll feel a wave of relaxation. Just try out a few statements until one gives you that surge of well-being.

What is your new approach to mood?

Your approach statement is a sensible plan for how you will deal with your emotions. Construct a statement that is brief and clear. Here are some ideas for your new approach to mood.

The Know Your Number Approach

You can keep it straightforward and brain-based, and simply check your number and use the tools.

There is no need to recreate the wheel here. My approach is to know my number and spiral up. Whether I'm flirting with depression, anxiety, or numbness, this approach takes me to Brain State 1.

My approach is to check in and use the tools. That way I can prevent my Mood Circuit from being activated or, if it's activated and I don't feel like using my Power Grind In, I can spiral up out of it.

Know Your Number Approach Examples
• Check my brain state.
• Use the tools.
• Spiral up to Brain State 1.

The Words I Need to Hear Approach

The thinking brain is our internal overseer, the good parent within. The circuits in the emotional brain are the kids. If a parent states the words a child most needs to hear in that moment, stress vanishes. This works best with circuits that are stored in the 3rd Drawer, as our thinking brain function is good enough to come up with those words.

My Mood Circuit is mild, stored in the 3rd Drawer, so if I gently tell myself that I am loved, and I am not in danger, that helps. I use a nurturing inner voice. I am cultivating that as part of my practice.

Words I Need to Hear Approach Examples
• Say the words that I need to hear.
• Tell myself, "I am creating joy in my life!"
• Talk to myself with a nurturing inner voice.

The Listen to My Body Approach

When a Mood Circuit is activated, our thinking brain cannot connect to the emotional brain. What do we most need? To reconnect! This approach of grounding ourselves with body awareness can be highly effective.

When my anxiety circuit is activated, I go right to Brain State 5. I use the 5 PLUS Tool which is really about rocking, breathing, and stroking. I was raised by a mother who was perpetually at Brain State 5. I acquired her set point. I like being grounded in my body to start the process. I can use the tools after that, if I want.

Listen to My Body Approach Examples
• Rock gently back and forth. • Focus on my breathing. • Stroke my body and soothe myself.

The Meet My Need Approach

The last approach is to wire into our brain the drive to meet the original need for safety, love, comfort, or pleasure. It's a simple approach because you bypass any plan for processing emotions and zero in on the underlying need.

That's the ticket! I tell myself to meet my basic need. If my need is comfort, I'll comfort myself. If my need is safety, I'll connect to the safe place inside me.

Meet My Need Approach Examples
• Meet my true need, rather than going numb. • Get my safety from inside me, not from a bad mood. • Get my love from spiraling up, not from staying stuck. • Comfort myself by feeling my feelings. • Feast on natural pleasures. • Bring to mind my reward for creating joy.

Where is your circuit stored?

Keep in mind where your circuit is stored. You may not be sure, but if the mood comes on slowly and/or is moderate, not extreme, it's probably in a higher drawer in the brain. Your thinking brain is functioning better, so you can use longer statements that are more abstract, such as: "know my number and use a tool to spiral up to One." What if that circuit is stored lower in the brain, activating so much stress that the neocortex is offline? A short, choppy, commanding statement is more effective, such as "STOP! CHECK MY NUMBER!"

Which reward matters most to you?

In choosing your reward, be practical. It takes work to switch off an unbalanced mood. In the moment that it is triggered, which of the rewards is so compelling that you would use your Power Grind In rather than letting the reptile take control and replay the old wire?

The Mood Circuit Imagine

Refine your Power Grind In for Mood by imagining a situation in which you would be likely to use it!

Relax: Set whatever limits are necessary to create privacy for yourself. Settle into a comfortable spot and begin to relax. Focus your attention on your body and your breathing. Breathe in through your nose and out through your mouth or in any way that is comfortable and comforting to you. Then when you are ready, begin to imagine.

Imagine: See yourself walking through your day, naturally moving through the whole range of brain states and living your life in a way that works for you at the time. Know that it is all perfect, no matter what, because your emotional brain is firing just the circuits that are there. Every good feeling you have is the firing of a circuit, and a reminder of how rewarding that wire feels. And every painful moment is the firing of a circuit that is reminding you through the language of stress, hurtful sensations, and negative emotions, that a wire is activated and primed for rewiring. This is the nature of the always-perfect emotional brain. Take a deep breath and continue to see yourself move through your day.

Now bring to mind a moment when your Mood Circuit has been activated. See that wire firing and your brain triggering that mood. Take a few moments and be aware of where you are . . . who is around you . . . how your body feels . . . and the thoughts that appear in your mind. Notice what you do . . .

Next, imagine words appearing in your mind that tell you to connect with yourself. Once you have those words in mind, take a few deep breaths. Now use those words. Tell yourself to connect to the deepest part of yourself.

Last, imagine words appearing in your mind that tell you how to process your emotions. What is your new approach to processing your feelings? What approach would work for you in that moment? Stay focused on that image of yourself in that scene, and the words that instruct you to use your new approach to processing your emotions.

Finally, bring to mind the reward that would make connecting to yourself and using this new approach worth the effort. Would it be Sanctuary, Authenticity, Vibrancy, Integrity, Intimacy, Spirituality, or Freedom? Please take all the time you need to imagine this scene and the words of your transformation statement. Use these discoveries to help you construct your transformation statement on the checklist at the end of this chapter.

The Power Grind In
(Counts as 10 Grind Ins)

Stage	Statements
1 SLOW	I can NOT get my safety from worrying.
2 RAMP UP	*That's ridiculous!* I can NOT get safety from worrying. How absurd. Worrying will NOT make me safe. *That's ridiculous!* NO WAY will worrying make me safe!
3 JOY	I get my safety from connecting inside, using the tools, and getting to One. My reward? Vibrancy. I get my safety from connecting inside, using the tools, and getting to One. My reward? *Vibrancy!* I get my safety from connecting inside, using the tools, and getting to ONE! My reward? VIBRANCY!

Sometimes your Power Grind In will change as you use it. If it does, update it, but then lock it in again, as repeating the same words, rather than varying them, is more effective in encoding and strengthening a new circuit.

I can . . . NOT . . . get . . . my . . . protection . . . from . . . hostility . . . That's ridiculous! I can NOT get my protection from hostility. Being hostile is not going to work. I can NOT get protection from hostility. I get protection from checking in and connecting to the love inside me. My reward: Sanctuary. I get protection from checking in and connecting to the love inside me. My reward: Sanctuary. I get REAL protection from checking in and connecting to the love inside me. My reward: Sanctuary!

I'm going to use my Power Grind In for Mood when I go to visit my mother. I know it will come up because she has a self-pity wire and so do I. It is, "I get my safety from feeling sorry for myself for everything that goes wrong." That's ridiculous! I cannot get my safety from feeling sorry for myself. That is absurd. No way is that true. I get my safety from checking in and using the tools to get to Brain State 1. My rewards? Sanctuary and Vibrancy.

Use the checklist on the next page to help you construct your Power Grind In for Mood, then use it as a Power Grind In (1 - slow negation, 2 - ridicule statements, and 3 - transform statements. Use your Food Grind In and your Mood Grind In through the day. Have fun with them!

At this point you have constructed two Power Grind Ins. Let's move forward with another lifestyle reset, then tackle the Love Circuit. Stay the course. The best is yet to come!

The Rewiring Checklist
Day 3. Transform Your Mood Circuit

After activating my Mood Circuit by stating my unreasonable expectation, I paused until I was at Brain State 3. Then I transformed it:

- **SLOW**

  I can NOT get my _____ from _____.

- **RAMP UP**

  That's ridiculous! I can NOT get my _____ from _____.

- **JOY**

I get my: _____ from:

CONNECT	APPROACH	REWARD
☐ Connecting with myself	☐ Checking my brain state	☐ Sanctuary
☐ Checking in	☐ Using the tools	☐ Authenticity
☐ Connecting to my body	☐ Getting to ONE!	☐ Vibrancy
☐ Taking a deep breath	☐ Feeling emotionally alive!	☐ Integrity
☐ Staying connected	☐ NOT numbing out!	☐ Intimacy
☐ Honoring my feelings	☐ Feeling my feelings	☐ Spirituality
☐ Connecting inside	☐ Using A+ Anger	☐ Freedom
☐ Being aware of my body	☐ NOT judging my feelings	
☐ Knowing my number	☐ Bringing up a nurturing inner voice	
☐ The deepest part of me	☐ Telling myself, "I am creating JOY in my life!"	
☐ Being present	☐ Using my brain's natural pathway from stress to joy	
☐ Other _____	☐ Other _____	

I transformed it: 50 75 100 125 150 200 _____ times.

Success Check Day 15

- **Daily Success**

☐ I continued my Joy Practice with 10 Check Ins and 10 Joy Points.

☐ I transformed my Mood Circuit and created my Power Grind In.

☐ I made one or more community connections for support with transforming my circuit.

- **Did I pass the Success Check?   YES   NO**

If you did not, stay with this activity for one more day, then move on.

- **My Amazing Learning:**

_____

- **My Biggest Accomplishment:**

_____

- **My Biggest Challenge:**

_____

Great Work!

You have completed Day 15 of The Joy Challenge.
Your next step is Day 16. Lifestyle Reset #3
Joy Lunch and Balancing Sleep.

Day 16. Lifestyle Reset #3
Joy Lunch and Balancing Sleep

Lunch matters, and so does sleep. Today we will upgrade both, and use a healthy lifestyle to experience a new zest for life.

Why

From this point on in this book, start resetting your lifestyle. Lifestyle has a huge impact on stress and pleasure. Each use of the tools strengthens the Joy Circuits and weakens the Stress Circuits. Why not make it easier to be at One by adding lifestyle changes, so that we can move up our set point more rapidly? A high set point keeps the Stress Triangle from being activated. It creates a healthier chemical environment, which is essential for ending overeating and achieving natural, lasting weight loss.

Honor Your Need for Natural Pleasure
- Savor a healthy Joy Lunch.
- Sleep well for eight hours.
- Track your progress in creating joy.

A Joy Lunch sustains our productivity

Our hunter-gatherer ancestors had their largest meal at lunch. This is why you've probably noticed that there are a lot of growling stomachs around midday.

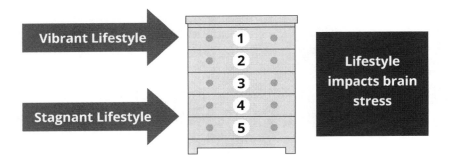

After eating a high-protein healthy breakfast, your energy will be solid, your blood sugar strong for four to six hours. The Joy Lunch emphasizes Joy Foods to stop insulin from overshooting and causing the cravings and hunger that block our freedom. Drink plenty of water and enjoy your mental acuity and good judgment. Eat lunch when you are hungry. Eat mainly Joy Foods, particularly fiber foods (vegetables and fruits), healthy fats (oils, avocados, and nuts) and lean protein (chicken, fish, lean meats, and eggs). Have agrarian foods if you like, as they are whole foods and many people do well on them. Have Stress Foods if you need them. Too much of the processed foods or agrarian foods can make for a sleepy afternoon, so be sure to stop eating when your hunger fades.

Your mind stays clearer, your relationships stay more connected, and your energy stays strong all afternoon. By evening you have enough stamina and energy to create a pleasurable evening, an Evening at One.

Why insulin matters!

Eating Joy Foods can stop the overshooting of
insulin and the resulting blood sugar low.
It reduces hunger and cravings!

"I eat Joy Foods. I want freedom in my life."

Sleep is like food for the brain

If you do not sleep well or long enough, the work you do during the day to check in and rewire circuits is largely flushed away at night. Sleep is when the brain consolidates the learning we have done during the day and locks it into long-term memory.

The better your sleep habits, the lower your levels of the stress hormone cortisol, so you are less apt to trigger brain glitches. By developing the habit of sleeping long and well, you can alter two important hormones: ghrelin and leptin. As these hormones change, they stop causing food cravings and constant hunger, which can be a relief for the 70 percent of us who are challenged by weight issues.

Changing sleep patterns is not easy, but sleep is so important to brain stress, that finding a way to get enough sleep is worth it. Do Cycles, get coaching, talk to your doctor, do whatever you need to find a healthy sleep pattern that works for you!

How

First, plan your Joy Lunch and Balancing Sleep. Check off ideas on the next page, then use them. Feel unmotivated or stalled? That's not a problem. Use your Power Grind In or the Cycle Tool!

The situation is . . . I eat Stress Foods for lunch, and I don't like Joy Foods. I like Stress Foods. What I'm most stressed about is . . . I have to change. I feel angry that . . . I have to change. I can't stand it that . . . I have to change. I HATE IT that . . . I have to change. I feel sad that . . . I have to change. I feel afraid that if I don't get my Stress Foods, I will fall apart. I feel afraid that if I cannot have my Stress Foods, I will die. (That's ridiculous!) I feel guilty that I am so rigidly tied to my Stress Foods. Of course I am rigidly tied to my Stress Foods, because I get my existence from eating Stress Foods! That rings true. My Food Circuit is still alive and well in my brain. I . . . can . . . NOT . . . get . . . my existence . . . from Stress Foods. That's ridiculous! I cannot get my existence from Stress Foods. That will never work. That's completely ridiculous! I get my existence from . . . connecting to the deepest part of myself . . . and eating foods that make me strong. My reward? Vibrancy. I get my existence from connecting to the deepest part of myself and eating foods that make me strong. I get my existence from CONNECTING to the deepest part of myself and eating foods that make me STRONG. YES! Okay, now I'm ready to eat my Joy Lunch!

The situation is . . . I watch videos until midnight and don't get enough sleep. What I'm most stressed about is . . . I have to shut off the light at 10:30 at the latest. What I'm most stressed about is . . . that I have to do something I don't want to do. I feel ANGRY that I have to do something I don't want to do. I can't stand it that I have to set limits with myself. I HATE it that I have to say "no" to myself. I HATE THAT!!! I feel sad that . . . I can't do whatever I want to do. I feel afraid that . . . I am not lovable. I feel guilty that . . . I don't take better care of myself. I expect myself to do the best I can to turn off the light earlier. Positive, powerful thought? I can do that. I can try. The essential pain? It takes work. The earned reward? Integrity, doing the right thing. What do I need? I need to be gentle with myself. This is hard for me. I need to turn the light off earlier. Do I need support? Yes, I will set the alarm at 10:00 to remind me, and I will ask my connection buddy to call me at that time to remind me. If I do both, it might work!

After you plan your Joy Lunch and Balancing Sleep and do as many Cycles as needed to follow through with joy and purpose, then take The Joy Inventory again. Compare your scores to your baseline scores and reflect on your amazing learnings.

Joy Lunch Ideas

- ☐ Emphasize lean protein, healthy fats, and fiber to boost productivity.
- ☐ If you need Stress Foods, have them without guilt.
- ☐ If you cannot control the type of food you eat, choose half portions.
- ☐ In restaurants, order by ingredients – "I want greens with chicken on top."
- ☐ Eat only when you are hungry.
- ☐ Choose salads topped by a protein source, drizzled with olive oil.
- ☐ Eat half a deli sandwich and bring the other half home for dinner.
- ☐ Drink four glasses of water or more during the workday.
- ☐ Keep healthy snacks on hand: nuts, fruit, a piece of chicken, olives . . .
- ☐ Bring a sack lunch to eat when you are hungry.
- ☐ If you overeat at lunch, check in three times in the early afternoon.
- ☐ Reward yourself with "dessert" after lunch – go outside and move!

Balancing Sleep Ideas

- ☐ Consider your relationship with sleep as important.
- ☐ Learn to calm and quiet yourself – it is a developmental task.
- ☐ Get enough exercise during the day so your body is tired.
- ☐ Do not eat or exercise for two hours before sleep.
- ☐ Stop use of all technology an hour before sleep.
- ☐ Overcome problems: snoring, uncomfortable bed, body pain . . .
- ☐ Make your bedroom dark and cool.
- ☐ Use natural sleep triggers, such as reading, a bath, or lovemaking.
- ☐ Check in and spiral up before going to sleep.
- ☐ Conclude your day with three Joy Points.
- ☐ If you awaken in the night, consider it a Moment of Opportunity.
- ☐ Do Power Grind Ins or use the tools until you to drift off to sleep.

The Joy Inventory

Needs

In the last week, how often did you meet each of your basic needs?

Purpose
    1 = Rarely   2 = Sometimes   3 = Often   4 = Very Often

Pleasure
    1 = Rarely   2 = Sometimes   3 = Often   4 = Very Often

Comfort
    1 = Rarely   2 = Sometimes   3 = Often   4 = Very Often

Love
    1 = Rarely   2 = Sometimes   3 = Often   4 = Very Often

Safety
    1 = Rarely   2 = Sometimes   3 = Often   4 = Very Often

Total Needs Score _____

Rewards

In the last week, how often did you experience these rewards?

Sanctuary: Peace and power from within
    1 = Rarely   2 = Sometimes   3 = Often   4 = Very Often

Authenticity: Feeling whole and being genuine
    1 = Rarely   2 = Sometimes   3 = Often   4 = Very Often

Vibrancy: Healthy with a zest for life
    1 = Rarely   2 = Sometimes   3 = Often   4 = Very Often

Integrity: Doing the right thing
    1 = Rarely   2 = Sometimes   3 = Often   4 = Very Often

Intimacy: Giving and receiving love
    1 = Rarely   2 = Sometimes   3 = Often   4 = Very Often

Spirituality: Aware of the grace, beauty, and mystery of life
    1 = Rarely   2 = Sometimes   3 = Often   4 = Very Often

Freedom: Common excesses fade
    1 = Rarely   2 = Sometimes   3 = Often   4 = Very Often

Total Rewards Score _____

Connection

In the last week, how often did you connect in this way?

Being aware that I can create joy in my life
    1 = Rarely   2 = Sometimes   3 = Often   4 = Very Often

Choosing to create a moment of joy
    1 = Rarely   2 = Sometimes   3 = Often   4 = Very Often

Spiraling up from stress to joy
    1 = Rarely   2 = Sometimes   3 = Often   4 = Very Often

Enjoying sensory pleasures
    1 = Rarely   2 = Sometimes   3 = Often   4 = Very Often

Appreciating the joy of eating healthy
    1 = Rarely   2 = Sometimes   3 = Often   4 = Very Often

Feeling the joy of releasing extra weight
    1 = Rarely   2 = Sometimes   3 = Often   4 = Very Often

Feeling love for myself
    1 = Rarely   2 = Sometimes   3 = Often   4 = Very Often

Feeling love for others
    1 = Rarely   2 = Sometimes   3 = Often   4 = Very Often

Feeling love for all living beings
    1 = Rarely   2 = Sometimes   3 = Often   4 = Very Often

Total Connection Score _____

The Joy Inventory Summary

Category	Baseline Score	Current Score	Progress	Joy Range
Needs	_____	_____	_____	15 to 20
Rewards	_____	_____	_____	21 to 28
Connection	_____	_____	_____	27 to 36
Total	_____	_____	_____	63 to 84

What is your amazing learning about your needs?

_____

What is your amazing learning about your rewards?

_____

What is your amazing learning about your connection?

_____

Success Check Day 16

- **Daily Success**

☐ I continued my Joy Practice with 10 Check Ins and 10 Joy Points.

☐ I reset my lifestyle in these five ways: Exercise, Joy Breakfast, Sanctuary Time, Joy Lunch, and Balancing Sleep.

☐ I made one or more community connections for support with my lifestyle reset.

- **Did I pass the Success Check?   YES   NO**

If you did not, stay with this activity for one more day, then move on.

- **My Amazing Learning:**

_____

- **My Biggest Accomplishment:**

_____

- **My Biggest Challenge:**

_____

Congratulations!

**You have completed Day 16 of Joy Challenge.
Your next step is Day 17. Discover Your Love Circuit.**

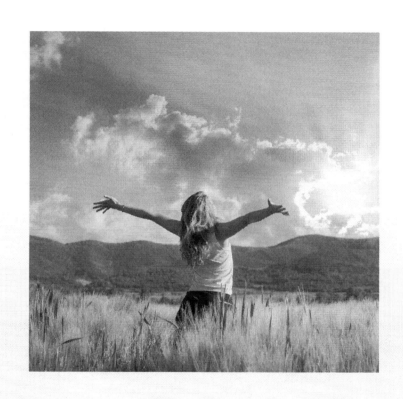

Release Weight

Day 17. Discover Your Love Circuit

You have stayed with the challenge! Congratulations. Now you'll build on your success by connecting even more deeply with yourself. As you feel intense love for yourself, releasing weight becomes a joy. Out of self-love comes less stress and the unconscious mind begins activating a drive to release extra weight. The easiest way to deepen that love is to rewire two circuits: the Love Circuit and the Body Circuit.

We'll start with the Love Circuit that changes how we conduct our relationships, neither merging with others nor distancing from them. Finding that sweet spot of staying connected to yourself, but aware of the feelings and needs of others, is the pathway to experiencing more love in your life.

The Love Circuit

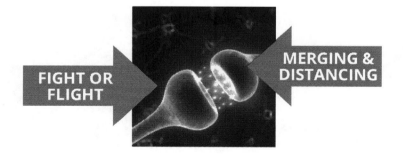

Why

We are mammals, and for all mammals, love is our first survival priority. We evolved to have such large heads to make room for conscious thought. That meant that our very existence depended upon creating loving connection to others, particularly during the first years of life. Even as adults, we have a strong love drive and much of our health and happiness is dependent upon being able

155

to keep our own boundary so we do not neglect or abuse ourselves, yet can give love to others. This is the most complex task that the brain takes on, and the one we are most apt to fail at!

The two survival circuits which cause us challenges in loving relationships are the drive to merge with others, losing ourselves in them and abandoning ourselves, and the drive to distance from others, becoming overly absorbed in ourselves and abandoning others. Both patterns are responsible for our deepest hurts, and the rewiring of these circuits so that we can be separate but close is often our greatest source of joy.

Love Circuits	Examples
Merging	rescuing, people pleasing, seeking validation, indulging others, denying my own needs, being the victim, being needy, being overly available, relentlessly seeking others, making everyone else happy
Distancing	hiding, judging, persecuting, criticizing, neglecting others, rejecting others, abusing others, putting up walls, manipulating, objectifying, ignoring their needs, taking too much, being sought by others, disappearing

The goal of these three days is for you to find the merging or distancing wire that blocks you from giving and receiving love. Then you will develop a Power Grind In that provides immediate deactivation of the drive to merge or distance. With repeated use over time, the same Power Grind In transforms the Love Circuit. The new circuit stops merging and distancing and activates a drive to be intimate, staying close but retaining our own essential boundary.

The Brain and Love Circuits
MERGING The prefrontal cortex attunes excessively to the emotional brain of the other person. We abandon ourselves.
DISTANCING The prefrontal cortex attunes excessively to our own emotional brain. We abandon others.

What does merging look like?

How do you know if you have a Merge Circuit? You won't be able to tell when stress is low. When we're running wires that are activated by the neocortex, we can easily connect with others. We get our survival needs – our safety, protection, power, nurturing, and existence – from the emotional connection between our thinking and feeling brains.

However, in stress, one fundamental brain function changes. Our prefrontal cortex stops attuning to our emotional brain and instead excessively focuses on the emotional brain of another. If we could just get something from them, we would be fine. We forget about our fundamental aloneness, that we are responsible for taking care of our own basic needs. We look for them to do it for us. We borrow their functioning.

If two people with Merge Circuits are in a committed relationship, and are chronically merged, the implicit agreement is that each will take care of the other. That way neither person will evolve beyond the circuits they downloaded from their parents. Neither one must grow.

My husband and I love each other very much. We feel love for each other, but we are excessively close. I don't set limits with him and he doesn't set limits with me. After dinner, he disappears into the kitchen and I can hear him grazing in the fridge. I shop on the internet, drink too much wine, and go to sleep early.

Even one person with a Merge Circuit in a relationship or family can block the system's emotional evolution. The purpose of relationships is to support each other's development, giving warm nurturing, emotional honesty, and effective limits. Sometimes friends won't do that for us; only those who really love us will! The Merge Circuit makes us so reactive to another person that we cannot tolerate allowing them to experience the pain that they need in order to grow.

I cannot stand it when my daughter is upset. I get an instant stomach ache and feel like I am going to die. I coddle her and obsess about how to prevent her from having all that pain. She is now 28 years old and is so adversity deficient that she has the maturity of a 12-year-old.

Merge Circuit Examples

- I get my safety from you.
- I get my security from rescuing you.
- I get my power from pleasing you.
- I get my safety from your approval.
- I get my power from not upsetting you.

What about distancing?

How do you know if you have a Distancing Circuit? In stress, your prefrontal cortex stops attuning to the emotional brain of others. It's not that you do not care, but your brain shuts down awareness of others as if your life depended on it. We forget about our fundamental need to emotionally connect with others. We don't know how they feel or what they need. In fact, without emotional connection, all we care about is getting what we want when we want it, without regard to the needs of others or our own need for connection in the longer term.

If two people with Distancing Circuits are in a committed relationship, and chronically disengaged, the implicit agreement is that each will take care of themselves. That way neither person will evolve beyond their comfort zone from childhood.

My partner and I are very busy people and we care about each other, but we live our own lives, perhaps to a fault. I am not a nurturing person so it doesn't bother me, and he has never been emotional. We are both addicted to our work and our relationship is functional. Yet our lack of closeness shows up in our sex life and in a sense that something is missing.

Like merging, even one person in a relationship or family with a Distancing Circuit can change the growth trajectory of the individuals involved. The Distancing Circuit makes us so unresponsive to another person's feelings and needs that we do not disrupt their circuits because we are not that impacted by them. We can either avoid conflict for decades or use high drama and conflict as a smokescreen that keeps real change from happening.

My husband and I are happily coupled, but he ran up over $100K of debt by investing in a start-up business with a partner who activated his Merge Circuit. It frustrated me that he is so irresponsible with money. I don't bring it up because I start judging him, and we have big blow-ups, then I go back to overspending and overeating.

Distancing Circuit Examples
• I get my security from putting up walls.
• I get my safety from hiding.
• I get my power from neglecting you.
• I get my protection from persecuting you.
• I get my existence from ignoring your needs.

The Seesaw – Merging AND Distancing

Most of us have both types of circuits. We switch circuits or seesaw between them to both merge and distance. Sometimes we lose ourselves in another, then feel hurt enough to distance. This is very common.

The Love Circuit Seesaw

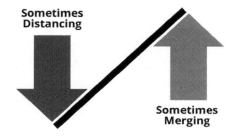

My unconscious mind activates merging with Katie, my younger daughter, who is four. My entire being wants to rescue her from all pain. My son, who is 10 and a carbon copy of my husband's dad, brings out my Distancing Circuit.

Many people are raised with one type of Love Circuit, and when they tire of the stress and loneliness it causes, they switch to the other.

My mother was a merger and so was every woman in my family. I'm not sure of my dad's circuits, but I stopped merging after I married a distancer who was depressed and drained my resources.

Rewiring Love Circuits – the new frontier of neuroplasticity

Until 10 years ago, the Stress Circuits that control emotional connection were thought to be hardwired. Now we know that they are plastic and open to change.

The idea that you can do the work in this book and attack an unwanted Merge or Distancing Circuit is nothing less than revolutionary. There is mounting evidence which suggests that we have the power to change our attachment styles. The most important research is that of Joseph LeDoux and Elizabeth Phelps who demonstrated our power to change our emotional circuitry. Also, the research of attachment scientist Phillip Shaver, from University of California, Davis, demonstrates that emotional connection is learned. In fact, 70 percent of our emotional connection style in stress can be predicted by our mother's attachment style. That connection appears to be environmental, not genetic.

Studies by Michael Meaney, from Montreal's McGill University, overturned the concept that genetics determine attachment style. He demonstrated in an elegant series of studies on rats (which are remarkably similar to humans) that even among offspring that had been birthed to stressed-out mothers (and so shared their genetics and in-utero experience of stress), if put in a nurturing environment, the rats evidenced signs of a secure connection.

Getting into the 5th Drawer

How do we rewire the way we connect? The traditional way is to seek psychotherapy. A supportive relationship can be helpful. Another way is to find love. Loving relationships heal. However, we tend to find partners who are at our set point, so if our set point is in stress, our partner will have either Merge or Distancing Circuits or both.

The EBT solution is to keep our sense of humor and appreciate that if we've had stress, we have a few of these circuits of disconnection. Let's go after those circuits, begin to raise our set point, and bring upgraded wires to our relationships. In the best of all worlds, we target and change a wire that is in the 5th Drawer. It's the most disruptive. Just bring to mind the relationship that bothers you the most and use the Stop a Trigger Cycle to discover it. Always start by complaining, and be certain to use A+ Anger to unlock that circuit.

The Travel Back experience

Sometimes the brain activates an old memory so that you can change it by using your imagination. Every time a circuit is activated, the hippocampus reconsolidates it, shifting it to long-term memory with alterations based on that experience. We are always updating our wiring.

When you do a deep Cycle – using A+ Anger and getting well into the 5th Drawer – right as you are discovering the circuit ("Of course I would do that, because my unreasonable expectation is . . . ") an image from the time the circuit was encoded might appear. If it does, you can "travel back" to that time and re-experience it.

The Travel Back Experience

- Do a Cycle about any deep hurt and be sure to use A+ Anger.
- Hope for an "unlocking moment" to discover circuits in the 5th Drawer.
- After finding the unreasonable expectation, focus on the place in your body that you experience the most stress.
- Relax and say, "I have felt that before." Allow your mind to travel back.
- Notice images that appear and settle on one of them. See yourself in that image, and feel love for yourself.
- If you like, imagine yourself as you are now, stepping into that image and giving your past self whatever you needed at that time to feel safe.
- Feel the glow in your body. You are wiring into your brain a secure connection to yourself.

You can imagine how you might have responded differently in that situation or reach a depth of understanding of yourself that can be profound. This can change the circuit and can provide a "reattachment" experience. Most faulty circuits cause us to disconnect from ourselves, and that broken connection is embedded in our circuitry, making it challenging to see ourselves, feel our feelings, and listen to ourselves. This reconnection heals us and is among the deepest work we do in EBT. Experience this solo, or with the support of friends, family members, connection buddies, or an EBT provider.

The nature of circuits – we can change our reality

Why does the Travel Back work? It's the nature of neural circuits. We think we are experiencing reality, but our reality is the experience that the activation of circuits delivers to us. As we change our circuits, we change our reality.

How do we travel back? We complain about a situation in our lives, such as a relationship. Those thoughts activate legions of wires stored in our unconscious mind. We notice activations of sensations and emotions in our body triggered by those wires. By turning our attention to our body, we block the prefrontal cortex from the overthinking that curtails the force of our imaginal mind. We focus on our body sensations of stress, further targeting the most egregious circuit, the memory of an experience that encoded the strongest Stress Circuit. We allow our mind to travel back via the images formed by the memories and one memory triggers another and another.

For example, the wire of an alarming scene of feeling invisible can trigger another wire that elicits feelings of being invisible, even though the people and situations were vastly different. Traveling back gives us a pathway to changing the root memory, as our mind seeks to find the deepest hurt. By discovering it we more fully activate the memory, and that activation gives us the power, using our consciousness, to choose to intervene by imagining, and to update that wire.

We change the wire by choosing to see our present selves enter into the image and say or do whatever our younger selves needed to avoid or minimize harm. The actual circuit, now updated, is reconsolidated by the hippocampus so that our reality changes.

I was using the Cycle Tool to find my Love Circuit and complaining about my boyfriend who is volatile. I arrived at the unreasonable expectation which is I get my safety from distancing from and judging him. Suddenly, I had this pit in my stomach. I realized that I was in the 5th Drawer and had unlocked a strong fear memory. It was a doozy of a Stress Circuit. I focused on my stomach and that stress, locked my mind into those sensations and said to myself – I've felt this way before. I allowed my mind to travel back and bring up images, each one leading to another that happened still earlier in my life. In about 30 seconds an image appeared that must have been from when it was encoded. I could see myself in the living room of our apartment and my dad booming his rant. I was so scared and distancing from him and judging him. It was how I emotionally survived that incident. I could see myself and I felt love for myself. The oddest part was that I chose to imagine me, the adult I am now, taking charge and entering the image to comfort her. I told her that she didn't have to judge him or distance emotionally. She could scream at him to stop or leave the room or get help from another adult. She could use her power without needing to judge or distance. The experience was a turning point for me in raising my set point. It was a reset.

Discover Your Love Circuit
I get my ____(need)____ from ____(merging or distancing)____ .

How

To discover your Love Circuit, bring to mind the relationship that causes you the most stress, either chronic stress that can mount up and create mindless eating, or chronic reliance on overeating to reduce stress or feel rewarded. Use the Stop a Trigger Cycle one or more times until you discover the unreasonable expectation that would make it perfectly reasonable for you to overeat.

Discover the hidden message of your Love Circuit

Use the same discovery process you have used for the first two circuits to find the words of the unreasonable expectation for your relationship wire. The words will follow the formula "I get my (need) from (merging or distancing)," as the wire is a false association made by the brain between a basic need and whatever relationship pattern we used in an effort to meet it.

Enjoy discovering the hidden message in your drive to merge or distance. As you discover and rewire this circuit, it will be far easier to find that sweet spot of loving connection in your relationships. That sweetness turns off the drive to overeat and activates the desire to eat healthy!

The Rewiring Checklist
Day 1. Discover Your Love Circuit

Say What Is Bothering You

- The situation is . . . (Complain about a relationship.)
- What I'm most stressed about is . . . (Say what bothers you the most about this relationship.)

Unlock the Circuit

- I feel angry that . . .
- I can't stand it that . . .
- I hate it that . . .

Discover the Hidden Message

- I feel sad that . . .
- I feel afraid that . . .
- I feel guilty that . . .
- OF COURSE I would do that, because my unreasonable expectation is . . .

I get my:	from:	
	MERGING	**DISTANCING**
☐ Safety		
☐ Love	☐ Others, not from myself	☐ Hiding
☐ Comfort	☐ Rescuing others	☐ Judging others
☐ Pleasure	☐ People pleasing	☐ Persecuting
☐ Purpose	☐ Seeking you	☐ Neglecting others
☐ Survival	☐ Others validating me	☐ Abusing others
☐ Existence	☐ Indulging others	☐ Shaming others
☐ Protection	☐ Denying my own needs	☐ Being sought by you
☐ Security	☐ Being the victim	☐ Putting up walls
☐ Power	☐ Making you happy	☐ Taking too much
☐ Nurturing	☐ Never making you angry	☐ Disappearing
☐ Other _____	☐ Other _____	☐ Other _____

Success Check Day 17

- **Daily Success**

☐ I continued my Joy Practice with 10 Check Ins and 10 Joy Points.

☐ I discovered my Love Circuit.

☐ I made one or more community connections for support with discovering my circuit.

- **Did I pass the Success Check?   YES   NO**

If you did not, stay with this activity for one more day, then move on.

- **My Amazing Learning:**

_____

- **My Biggest Accomplishment:**

_____

- **My Biggest Challenge:**

_____

Congratulations!

You have completed Day 17 of The Joy Challenge.
Your next step is Day 18. Negate Your Love Circuit.

Day 18. Negate Your Love Circuit

Let's weaken and break that circuit! Finding that sweet spot of connection in which you can give and receive love can become a habit. However, as long as a fight-or-flight drive obscures that sweet spot, we cannot strengthen our intimacy circuits. We get triggered to either distance or merge!

Definitely feel love for that circuit and do all the Cycles you need to do to grieve the losses it has caused. That Love Circuit was encoded because we did not feel safe. It was a default option when we were highly stressed and needing to find some way to connect!

I have a Merge Circuit and I turn into a different person when it is activated. I am so anxious, as if I want to crawl out of my own skin. That anxiety is enough to make anyone want to overeat. I come from a family of mergers and I've seen how merging hurts people. I want to clear that circuit.

Merging and Distancing:
These wires keep me from getting the love that I need.

Why

We clear this circuit because it blocks our capacity for love. We are on a mission now to support our mammalian brain in effectively connecting with other people. We need that warm glow of loving connection. What's more, merging is so stressful. When the switch flips from connecting with ourselves to abandoning ourselves to depend on the love, approval, or validation of others, our emotional evolution stops. Often we sense that we have regressed.

My daughters and I went to visit my mother and they pointed out to me how I change when I am around my mother. My mom treats me as if I do not exist, and my Merge Circuit obeys her expectations, not mine. It messages me, "Because your mother thinks she does not exist, then you do not exist." That wire triggers my mother's expectations to overpower my own. A glance at her face and I feel like I'm eight again. I don't want to endure this babyish anxiety the rest of my life, and I do not want to pass these wires along to my children and grandchildren.

Distancing is just as ineffective. What do we need? Emotional connection. Yet that distancing circuit tells us that we get our safety by disappearing, persecuting, judging, or hiding (just a few examples). When we distance, it's as if we have given up hope. We will never get the love we need, so why try? Distancing often triggers a lost, abandoned feeling and a drive for over-control. Depression or numbness often co-activate with the distancing wire.

When I was 12, my father, who really loved me, became uncomfortable with my changing body and distanced from me. I was devastated, and have been a distancer ever since. I have never grieved the loss of that sudden rejection. I need to rewire my Distancing Circuit and clear the emotional trash from that hurt.

How

Use the same negation process you used with your Food and Mood Circuits. First, stress-activate the circuit to unlock it. The easiest way is to state the unreasonable expectation, such as: **"I get safety from making everybody happy all the time."** Then say, **"I can NOT get safety from making everybody happy all the time."** Again, state it very slowly at first, then ramp it up and ridicule the circuit. If you like, sing or dance or stomp when you are negating it. Making community connections helps tremendously. The more emotionally-charged the experience, the better the rewiring results.

	2 Stages of Negating a Love Circuit
SLOW	I . . . can . . . NOT . . . get . . . my . . . safety . . . from . . . people pleasing. I . . . can . . . NOT . . . get . . . my . . . safety . . . from . . . people pleasing. I . . . can . . . NOT . . . get . . . my . . . safety . . . from . . . people pleasing.
RAMP UP	That's totally ridiculous! I can NOT get safety from PEOPLE PLEASING. Pleasing everyone all the time does not make me safe. That's ridiculous! I can NOT get MY safety from pleasing everybody!

Example (All Grind In Clusters count as 10 Grind Ins)

SLOW

- I . . . can . . . NOT . . . get . . . SAFETY . . . from . . . judging others . . . (pause)
- I . . . can . . . NOT . . . get . . . SAFETY . . . from . . . judging others . . . (pause)
- I . . . can . . . NOT . . . get . . . SAFETY . . . from . . . judging others . . . (pause)
- I . . . can . . . NOT . . . get . . . SAFETY . . . from . . . judging others . . . (pause)
- I . . . can . . . NOT . . . get . . . SAFETY . . . from . . . judging others . . . (pause)

RAMP UP

- That's ridiculous! I can NOT get safety from judging!
- Judging does NOT make me safe.
- Judging people does NOT give me the safety that I need.
- That's ridiculous! I can NOT get my safety from JUDGING!
- Totally ridiculous! I can NOT get my safety from JUDGING!
- I CANNOT GET MY SAFETY from JUDGING PEOPLE!

Grieving is normal – Do 5 Cycles

Grieving takes as long as it takes! Do cycles in clusters of five. At this point, you may want to establish a Cycle Journal and write three pages of Cycles in it daily to deepen your EBT Practice. That's a great way to clear away the past and move forward with your life. This will be part of your EBT practice in the advanced courses.

Our relationship circuits are strong because they are encoded early in life. Updating any strong circuit will cause grieving. Even if that circuit harmed us a great deal, it's familiar to the reptilian brain. Changing it is a loss. Be very careful to do as much grieving as you need to do before negating this circuit. Use any and all of the Cycles. Clear away that emotional clutter so that you feel charged up and ready to negate this wire!

The situation is . . . my Love Circuit is merging. I people please. I have been trying to please my father since I was six years old. My mind is traveling back as I say that, and I can see my father. He encoded the wire that I had to please him, or I would be a goner. I would lose his approval. What I'm most stressed about is . . . My father didn't give me love. He made me disconnect from myself and do whatever I thought he wanted to do so that I could please him and feel safe. I feel angry that . . . he put that circuit in me. I can't stand it that . . . I am a big people pleaser. I hate it that . . . he did that to me. I HATE THAT!!!! I HATE THAT!!! . . . I feel sad that . . . I have merged . . . I feel afraid that . . . I will always disconnect from myself, feel intense anxiety, and people please. I feel guilty that . . . I didn't scream at him to stop making me into someone I wasn't and to just love me!!! OF COURSE I would not scream at him, because my unreasonable expectation is . . . I have no power. That rings true. I'm going to change that expectation! I do have power. I DO have power . . . OF COURSE I have power. I DO HAVE POWER. Yes I do. I have POWER and I'm going to use it . . . to bust this Love Circuit. Yahoo! I feel great . . . I'm going to negate that circuit now!

I think I merged early in my life, but at around the time I started high school, I encoded a distancing circuit. I drank and partied. I didn't care about anyone but myself. People liked me, but I didn't like myself, and that made me distance more. I didn't want anyone to see me – really know me – because they would reject me. The situation is . . . I have been distancing for decades now and what I'm most stressed about is . . . how much opportunity for happiness I lost. What I'm most stressed about is . . . how unhappy I have been because I have not built a family life. I am successful in my work but in love, I have not invested in relationships that satisfy me. What I'm most stressed about is . . . I do not have love in my life. I feel ANGRY that . . . I do not have love in my life. I can't STAND IT that . . . I am so lonely. I HATE it that . . . actually, I'm sad. I feel sad that . . . I have no friends . . . I feel afraid that . . . I'll continue to put up walls. I feel guilty that . . . I put up walls. OF COURSE I put up walls, because my unreasonable expectation is . . . I get my safety from people not rejecting me. OH MY GOSH. Under my Distancing Circuit is a Merge Circuit! Fascinating . . .

Let's add some Power Boosters

Continue to use the Power Boosters you have learned so far but add to them ways to share your Grind Ins with others. The brain experiences the Grind Ins differently when we are being seen, heard, and felt by another.

Power Boosters for your Love Circuit

- Grind it in whenever you sense you are distancing or merging.
- Say it to a Connection Buddy.
- Ask a family member or friend to listen to you grind it in.
- Post your Grind In on the EBT Community Forum Boards.
- Record yourself saying it, then listen to your recording.

The same way that when you fry your Food Circuit, you discover you actually LIKE healthy food, as you clear your Love Circuit, you will discover your natural capacity to give and receive love. The circuit is the problem. Let's tromp it!

The Rewiring Checklist
Day 2. Negate Your Love Circuit

I activated my Love Circuit by stating my unreasonable expectation, then paused until I was at Brain State 3. Then I negated it:

- **SLOW**

  I can NOT get my _____ from _____.

- **RAMP UP**

  That's ridiculous! I can NOT get my _____ from _____.

  I negated it: 50   75   100   125   150   200 _____ times.

I boosted the power of my Grind In (one or more ways):

- ☐ Grinding it in whenever I sense I'm distancing or merging

- ☐ Saying it to a Connection Buddy

- ☐ Asking a family member or friend to listen to me grind it in

- ☐ Posting my Grind In on the EBT Community Forum Boards

- ☐ Recording myself saying it, then listening to my recording

Success Check Day 18

● **Daily Success**

☐ I continued my Joy Practice with 10 Check Ins and 10 Joy Points.

☐ I negated my Love Circuit.

☐ I made one or more community connections for support with negating my circuit.

● **Did I pass the Success Check?   YES   NO**

If you did not, stay with this activity for one more day, and then move on.

● **My Amazing Learning:**

_____

● **My Biggest Accomplishment:**

_____

● **My Biggest Challenge:**

_____

Great Work!

You have completed Day 18 of The Joy Challenge.
Your next step is Day 19. Transform Your Love Circuit.

Day 19. Transform Your Love Circuit

Today you will create a Power Grind In for your Love Circuit. Whenever that urge to merge or that drive to distance shows up, you will zap it with your Power Grind In. Your natural capacity to give and receive love will appear!

This is your chance to rewrite your brain's script about how to love. The old circuit is damaged, weakened, and loosened up, so you have a wonderful opportunity to create a new way of relating to others. In turn, your healthy new wire will encode healthy new love wires in others.

I am so merged with my mother that I break out in an anxious sweat when she calls. Now my teenage daughter is showing the same anxiety about her boyfriend. I am stopping that merging with my mom and already, I can see the change in my daughter!

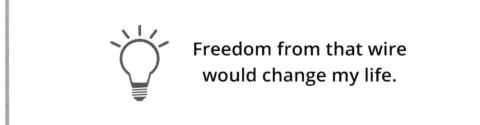

Freedom from that wire
would change my life.

Nobody showed me how to have a relationship. My mom and dad tolerated each other, but there was no passion. I connected with food and success. I found my passion in work, have two advanced degrees. Now is my time to try to find love. My first step is to crush my distancing circuit!

I'm happily married, but emotional honesty did not run in our family. I could be convinced that Mark and I have a perfect marriage, but I don't think I'd be binge eating after dinner if I felt safe being open with him. I want to transform my Love Circuit and embrace emotional honesty.

Why

The Power Circuit for Love is an extremely practical one. It solves many problems because most of our stress comes from relationship challenges. Change one unsatisfying relationship and your stress level can plummet. When stress is low, the remnants of that Food Circuit will not be activated! It's easier to stop stress eating.

My father-in-law is really gruff with me. I can't stand how he treats me, and when we'd go to his house, I'd always stuff myself with carbs. I used my Power Grind In before visiting him last weekend. I didn't merge. In fact, I told him that when he talks to me that way it scares me. He was shocked. Best of all, I didn't overeat. I had a good time visiting him.

I have not forgiven my mother for how stressed she was when she raised us. Yet I don't like myself when I avoid her. When she calls, I do not pick up the call and then head right for the freezer where I keep my ice cream stash. I have been using my Power Grind In. When she called this time, I picked up. We actually had a warm conversation, and I had no desire afterward to eat sweets.

Even better, as your natural capacity to give love to others – stopping short of neglecting or abusing yourself – kicks in, so does the power of oxytocin. This love chemical is a highly effective appetite suppressant. Giving yourself these chemical surges takes away the desire to stress eat.

My social anxiety doesn't bother me anymore and I owe that to my Power Grind In for Love. I'm finding myself really connecting with people, and feeling satisfied, as if I have eaten cake or bread, but I haven't. I think it's the oxytocin factor.

How

There are three parts to your new instruction to your brain about how to approach experiencing more loving connection in your life.

Connect: Tell yourself to connect with the deepest part of yourself. That connection – strong, loving, and wise – is the foundation of your ability to give and receive love.

Approach: State your approach to love. Try out different words until you find some that short-circuit merging and distancing and activate a healthy drive to give and receive love. Below are four approaches to this statement plus some examples and a visualization activity. Use them to construct your approach statement.

Reward: The reward is not always Intimacy! It can be any of the seven rewards, whichever is your motivating force. Some people stop merging for the reward of Integrity. Others want to stop distancing to intensify their Vibrancy. Some want to deepen their Spirituality. Still others want more love in their lives because they sense that without Intimacy, they will not let go of stress eating. Their reward is Freedom.

Where is your circuit stored?

Consider where your Love Circuit is stored. For example, **if your Love Circuit is activated gradually and moderately then it's probably in the 3rd Drawer**. A gentle reminder to give love, while stopping short of abuse or neglect, might be enough to help you not merge or distance. **If it is stronger or activates more rapidly, it's probably in the 4th Drawer**. Be more directive and quite specific. **If it activates an overwhelming drive to distance or merge, then it is in the 5th Drawer**. Don't hold back with the message of your Power Grind In. All 5 Circuits are survival circuits, the most extreme drives we have. Be commanding, as the reptile doesn't listen if we are not committed to having our way and expressing that forcefully!

My history has been merging with someone, and then when I couldn't stand the loss of control anymore, leaving them. The drives were really strong. I think my Merge Circuit is in the 4th Drawer and my Distancing Circuit in the 5th Drawer. I will go after my Distancing Circuit because it is in the 5th Drawer. Perhaps crushing that wire will weaken or clear my merge wire.

What is your new approach to relationships?

The reptilian brain needs directions, particularly when it comes to love. Choose an approach that helps you move toward intimacy as a personal skill, something you know how to do, a competency!

The Bolster Boundaries Approach

This approach works well if you are a merger, particularly someone whose urge to merge wire is stored in the 5th Drawer of the brain. This approach is so rewarding because setting limits, even having a Zero Tolerance Policy about neglect or abuse, can be highly effective. Decide what is "off limits" and make that your new approach to relationships.

I have a Zero Tolerance Policy for talking to my husband when he is at Brain State 5. I tell him that I can't hear him when he yells at me. And that I love him and will talk with him again later on. I do it lovingly and it's already made a change in our relationship.

The boundary I set is that I do not open my mouth and talk to my wife when I am overwhelmed (Brain State 5). I take a shower, go to bed, make a community connection, or watch sports on television, but I don't engage with her until I am at Brain State 3 or above. Our relationship is already becoming less volatile. My approach is NO TALKING until I am at Brain State 3 or above.

Bolster Boundaries Approach Examples

- Do not rescue people.
- Stop seeking validation from others.
- Do not accept neglect or abuse.
- Say how you feel and what you need.
- NO MERGING!

The Unconditional Love Approach

If you have a Distancing Circuit, this approach can be highly effective as it not only can short-circuit distancing but often improves the most common Mood Circuit associated with distancing: depression.

How do you use it? Just tell your reptilian brain that you are going to love, not judge. Be matter of fact! It's a policy switch! What if you do not have love to give? Use the tools. Spiral up to One and you'll have so much love to give that it will shock you. That's right! Abundant love. Then give some away. The giving of love manufactures even more love.

I am in abject terror at the thought of getting close to anyone. My Mood Circuit is to go numb and this wire is to judge, hide, or overwork. I can direct myself to love more. Something has to change. At this point, I do not like EBT. That must be my lizard brain revolting. EBT has me cornered and that's probably what it's going to take to get me to change.

Unconditional Love Approach Examples

- Do my best to give love.
- Feel compassion for others.
- NO DISTANCING!
- Ask how they feel and what they need.
- It's a policy. I love rather than judge.

The Finding the Sweet Spot Approach

If your Love Circuit is in a higher drawer in the brain, your prefrontal cortex can direct the emotional circuits in elegant ways. It can attune to your emotional brain and check how you feel and what you need, then attune to the emotional brain of another person and check how they feel and what they need. This "reading" by the brain enables us to shift our boundary rapidly. One moment we can have a tissue-paper-thin boundary when love is safe, and the next, a vault-thick boundary when there is danger. This keeps relationships vibrant, emotionally honest, and growing.

How do you find the sweet spot?

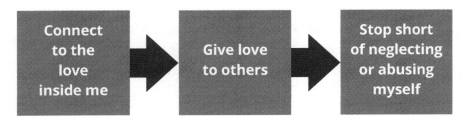

Connect to the love inside me → Give love to others → Stop short of neglecting or abusing myself

The sweet spot of love starts with feeling grounded in our own unconditional love for ourselves. At that point, we have enough love to give without triggering a 5 State. We start giving love without taking our fingers off the pulse of our own inner life. We stay connected to ourselves and enjoy giving love. However, we are always aware of our inner state. The moment giving that love is more than we can do without merging with the other person or triggering a strong desire to distance, we pull back somewhat. This is the dance of healthy intimacy. It is hard work, requires being present, and is the greatest joy of all.

Finding the Sweet Spot Approach Examples

- Give and receive love.
- Stay separate but close.
- Be emotionally honest.
- Get to One before speaking up.
- Give love stopping short of abusing or neglecting myself.

The fact that I have to find love inside me as a first step in intimacy is news to me. I thought I depended upon outside relationships for love. The fact that it starts with the love I have for myself changes a lot of things for me. I need to think about that!

The Meet My Need Approach

The last approach is to identify why the brain encoded your Love Circuit and be sure to meet that original need. It's a simple solution and can be quite effective.

My unmet need that caused my brain to encode a Merge Circuit was safety. I grew up in a family that was very chaotic. I didn't feel safe and didn't know what to do about it. I committed early to a friendship with David and eventually married him. That leftover unmet need of not knowing how to make myself safe remains. If I deal with my safety issues, my relationship might improve.

The unmet need that led my reptilian brain to encode distancing was comfort. I felt safe growing up and I had my mother's love, but never learned how to ground my life in basic comforts. The reason I don't date is that I wouldn't want to bring someone into my apartment. It is full of clutter. I want to learn how to develop a lifestyle that comforts me.

Meet My Need Approach Examples

- Meet my true need, rather than distancing or merging.
- Get my core safety from inside me, not from others.
- Get my basic love from myself, rather than from others.
- Comfort myself in healthy ways.
- Feast on healthy pleasures.
- Bring to mind my reward for not merging.
- Bring to mind my reward for not distancing.

The Love Circuit Imagine

Develop your transformation statement by using the brain's ability to activate circuits based on an Imagine. Use this visualization to generate, verify, or fine-tune the instructions your brain needs to transform your Love Circuit.

Relax: Create a situation in which you have privacy and will not be interrupted. Find a comfortable location for yourself and begin to relax. Focus your attention on your body and your breathing. Breathe in through your nose, out through your mouth, or in any way that is comfortable and comforting to you. When you are ready, begin to imagine.

Imagine: See yourself walking through your day, moving through the whole range of brain states and doing what you need to do. Notice your boundary changing, sometimes very thick for protection and sometimes quite thin allowing for the giving and receiving of love. Be aware that you have emotional range and your boundary varies to some degree.

Now see yourself about to encounter someone who is important to you and with whom you know for sure that your Merge or Distancing Circuit could be activated. Take a deep breath and continue to see yourself move through your day. See that wire about to fire. Take a few moments and be aware of where you are . . . who is around you . . . how your body feels . . . and the thoughts that appear in your mind. Notice what you do . . .

Last, imagine yourself taking out your Power Grind In and saying words to yourself . . . words that give you a clear instruction to connect with yourself. Then imagine words appearing in your mind to express the approach statement you need to hear. Take a few deep breaths . . . Notice that if you stay focused on your body, imagining that scene, the words will bubble up into your mind. Finally, which reward would motivate you to follow through and connect with yourself and use that approach? Would it be Sanctuary, Authenticity, Vibrancy, Integrity, Intimacy, Spirituality, or Freedom?

Please take all the time you need and then, use the upcoming checklist to record the transformation statement that feels right to you.

The Power Grind In for Love: Merging Example

Stage	Statements
1 SLOW	I can NOT get my safety from making people happy all the time.
2 RAMP UP	That's ridiculous! I can NOT get safety from making everyone happy all the time. That's ridiculous. I can NOT get safety from making everyone happy all the time!
3 JOY	I get my safety from connecting to myself and being emotionally honest with people. Reward: Authenticity. I get my safety from connecting to MYSELF and being emotionally honest with people. Reward: It's Authenticity. Yes I do! I GET my safety from connecting to myself and being emotionally honest. Reward: AUTHENTICITY!

The Power Grind In for Love: Distancing Example

Stage	Statements
1 SLOW	I can NOT get my safety from hiding.
2 RAMP UP	That's ridiculous! I can NOT get safety from hiding. That's ridiculous. I can NOT get safety from hiding.
3 JOY	I get my safety from connecting to the love inside me and showing up in people's lives. Reward: Integrity. I get my SAFETY from connecting to the love inside me and showing up in people's lives. Reward: Integrity. I get my safety from connecting to the love inside me and showing up in people's lives. Reward: Integrity!

When you're alone, you're in good company

As you rewire your Love Circuit, be sure to honor your need to strengthen your relationship with yourself. The first four Advanced EBT courses focus on building a secure base within. The rewards of Sanctuary, Authenticity, Vibrancy, and Integrity are fundamental to a secure attachment to self. With that base, we can nurture others more deeply and set limits with them, too. Also, we can heal from the past.

The healing process takes time, but we are born to heal because our circuits need to be updated to favor the survival of the species. We have the brain power to rewire emotional circuits encoded by hurtful experiences. Evolutionary biology uses positive and negative emotions to guide our development. According to the research of neuroscientist Antonio Damasio, we continue to experience the negative emotions triggered by our old hurts as gentle reminders to process them. When we do, the genome rewards us with the joy of "post-traumatic growth" which is a natural high like none other.

Each wire that we process holds a nugget of wisdom, an unreasonable expectation that becomes reasonable. Think of any trauma as the cause for a cluster of 5 Circuits forming in the brain, much like a rubber band ball. Each Cycle takes off one rubber band and at some point, we have gained so much wisdom from healing that the hurt, like the ball, is gone. It's quite common at that point to be grateful that we had the hurt because of the maturity and sense of purpose that come from the healing.

My Distancing Circuit triggered me to cheat on my partner, and then blocked me from really understanding how much hurt I had caused. For 11 years after that horrible time, I was numb and self-loathing. A year ago, I started using EBT and cycling through that experience. I went through every recollection, and circuit by circuit, I came to peace with what I did. I became far more empathetic and loving, and the sting of that hurt is gone.

Create your Power Grind In for Love

Please create the words of your Power Grind In that will guide your way in rewiring your Love Circuit. Grind it in 50 to 200 times today, so that your thinking brain strongly remembers it. Use the checklist that follows.

Once you've developed your Power Grind In, use it in daily encounters. Appreciate that you will break and transform that circuit during the second 30 days of this program. However, right now, use your Grind In as often as possible, at least four times per day.

Celebrate creating your second Power Grind In and prepare to move forward for a lifestyle reset and onward to your Body Circuit!

The Rewiring Checklist
Day 3. Transform Your Love Circuit

After activating my Love Circuit by stating my unreasonable expectation, I paused until I was at Brain State 3. Then I transformed it:

- **SLOW**

    I can NOT get my _____ from _____.

- **RAMP UP**

    That's ridiculous! I can NOT get my _____ from _____.

- **JOY**

I get my: _____ from:

CONNECT	APPROACH	REWARD
☐ Connecting with myself	☐ Giving and receiving love	☐ Sanctuary
☐ Checking in	☐ Being emotionally honest	☐ Authenticity
☐ Taking a deep breath	☐ Loving, not judging, others	☐ Vibrancy
☐ Being aware of myself	☐ Opening up, not distancing!	☐ Integrity
☐ Staying connected	☐ STOP merging with people!	☐ Intimacy
☐ Honoring my feelings	☐ NO MORE People Pleasing!	☐ Spirituality
☐ Connecting inside	☐ Being separate but close to others	☐ Freedom
☐ Listening to my body	☐ Having ZERO TOLERANCE (abuse or other)	
☐ Knowing my number	☐ Getting to One before I speak to others	
☐ The deepest part of me	☐ Feeling compassion for myself and others	
☐ Feeling my feelings	☐ Giving love stopping short of neglecting myself	
☐ Other _____	☐ Other _____	

I transformed it: 50   75   100   125   150   200 _____ times.

Success Check Day 19

- **Daily Success**

☐ I continued my Joy Practice with 10 Check Ins and 10 Joy Points.

☐ I transformed my Love Circuit and created my Power Grind In.

☐ I made one or more community connections for support with transforming my circuit.

- **Did I pass the Success Check?   YES   NO**

If you did not, stay with this activity for one more day, then move on.

- **My Amazing Learning:**

_____

- **My Biggest Accomplishment:**

_____

- **My Biggest Challenge:**

_____

Great Work!

You have completed Day 19 of The Joy Challenge.
Your next step is Day 20. Lifestyle Reset #4
Natural Pleasure Binge and Joy Dinner.

Day 20. Lifestyle Reset #4
Natural Pleasure Binge and Joy Dinner

Let's take back the night! Today you will plan and experience an Evening at One. You will meet your most important needs and experience an abundance of the natural pleasures of life.

Why

What happens after 4 p.m. is make-it-or-break-it for the quality of our lives, and for releasing extra weight. The prescription? Take back the night and stuff it with natural pleasures. Who knows what could happen?

To eat healthy all day, and then come home to rely on artificial pleasures and excesses, sets the stage for disrupting sleep, changing hormones, causing food hangovers, and blocking fat burning. The evening is the perfect time to pour on natural pleasures with gusto, because you will see results.

This morning I woke up hungry, which means I was releasing weight all night. Usually I have a food hangover. I woke up and said, "I am creating joy in my life!" and I meant it. I collected a Joy Point.

I did this with my wife and kids. The kids were calmer, sharing their toys. My wife and I had time to relax together. She played the guitar for the first time in a long time.

Take Back the Night
- Identify Your Deepest Needs.
- Determine Your Reward.
- Experience an Evening at One.

How

What I love about EBT is that it is so basic. Our brains are vastly different from one another when it comes to thoughts, but remarkably the same in terms of what rewards and satisfies us. We all have basic needs and when we meet them, we run Joy Circuits in the evenings.

Step 1. Identify your deepest needs

Let's stand back from the evening and identify our most fundamental needs. By the time the evening arrives, which needs will you have met and which ones will you want to start meeting in the evening?

Take Back the Night
Step 1. Identify Your Deepest Needs

Check off the unmet needs you will meet this evening:

☐ Safety   ☐ Love   ☐ Comfort   ☐ Pleasure   ☐ Purpose

Step 2. Determine your reward

To marshal the drive to effectively meet those needs, the brain's reward center must light up from feel-good chemicals. These chemicals come from tapping into the deeper rewards of life. Check in more deeply with yourself to determine which reward will take you up and over to meeting those needs.

Take Back the Night
Step 2. Determine Your Reward

Which reward will motivate you to meet these needs?

☐ Sanctuary   ☐ Authenticity   ☐ Vibrancy   ☐ Integrity

☐ Intimacy   ☐ Spirituality   ☐ Freedom

Step 3. Make your plan to take back the night

Pull out all the stops. Make this evening meet your needs. A cornerstone of this evening is a natural pleasures binge. See ideas that bring sensory pleasures and any other natural joys that our hunter-gatherer ancestors used. No technology. Nothing that uses substances, artificial pleasures, or addictive devices. Be a hunter-gatherer for one night and experience long-overlooked joys and an easy way to be at One.

Be sure to plan for support. If you have a circle of connection buddies, plan several connections with each of them. A one- to five-minute call boosts oxytocin, which quiets appetite and makes natural pleasures more satisfying. Also, invite family members and friends to "Take Back the Night" or share an "Evening at One" with you. Spend the evening together or connect by telephone so the richness of one another's voices activates your reward center. You can't have too much support with EBT! The emotional brain loves connection even more than artificial rewards!

Take Back the Night
Step 3. Experience an Evening at One
Check off what you plan to do:

ESSENTIAL

☐ A Natural Pleasure Binge
☐ A Joy Dinner
☐ Freedom from Artificial Pleasures

OPTIONAL

☐ Move in Joy
☐ Play
☐ Sanctuary Time
☐ Community Connections
☐ Sleep
☐ Emotional Connection
☐ Sensual Pleasure
☐ Sexual Pleasure
☐ Loving Companionship
☐ Spiritual Practices
☐ Social Activities
☐ Home/Life Upkeep
☐ Reading
☐ Caring for Others
☐ Altruistic Work

---

*What I need is **Safety**. I'm so tired when I get home that I know my blood pressure is up and I'm on the edge of quarreling with my wife or drinking too much. To encode wires that bring me safety I need to take 30 minutes of time alone in the garage. What reward would motivate me to do that? **Intimacy**. I want a loving evening, not one that goes south. I am on board for a Joy Dinner: steak, salad, and fruit. Will skip the scotch, but have one glass of wine (that's natural right?). I will go on a bike ride for my pleasure and see if my wife will play strip poker, like before we were married. That is my evening at One.*

*My need is for **Love**. I have a good paying job, but the office is very cold and my day is lonely. I am going to start taking five-minute breaks to make community connections, a couple in the morning and a couple in the afternoon, so I am not completely 5ish and feeling love-deprived by the time I come home. In the evening, I like having time alone (even though love is what I need). I live alone, have a cat, and am not ready to date. I have a neighbor friend I like and my strategy is to go out one night per week to a community event. My reward? It's **Integrity**. It's the right thing to stop being so cut off. My pleasure binge is going to be an evening basketball game with my neighbor, soaking in a hot tub, and eating fish with veggies, and strawberries. Technology is out. I'm going to have a ball!*

Natural Pleasure Binge Rules

The rules for the natural pleasure binge are simple: Do not do anything that our hunter-gatherer ancestors did not do. Our brain is set up for these natural pleasures so their potential to become Stress Circuits is low, and they do not bring artificial happiness, but a deep, natural joy! When doing them, you are MORE connected to yourself, not less! What a great way to live!

What about having a Joy Dinner?

That's easy. Be sure to have some lean protein, healthy fat, and plenty of fiber foods that are veggies or fruit. Eat agrarian foods if you like but skip the post-industrial-revolution foods ("Stress Foods"). Eat early enough in the evening that you can take a food rest for 12 hours minimum to clear excess glucose and glycogen from your system and perhaps burn up some triglycerides (fat). Your dessert – as many natural pleasures as you like!

Why ghrelin matters!

Stress increases ghrelin, the "start eating" hormone.
High ghrelin levels promote overeating in the evenings.

"I de-stress to reduce my ghrelin and stop overeating."

Freedom from Artificial Pleasures

This means freedom from technology: no phones, texting, computers, television, tablets, except using the phone for calling to connect with others. No devices or equipment that our hunter-gatherer ancestors did not have. No gambling, video games, or anything that has high addiction potential. This is your time to explore the natural pleasures of life.

Ideas for Your Natural Pleasure Binge

☐ Taking a long, hot shower

☐ Enjoying the sensory pleasure of sight – looking at the stars

☐ Playing with my dog or cuddling with my cat

☐ Enjoying the sensory pleasure of sound

☐ Drawing, painting, sculpting, or playing with clay

☐ Singing, dancing, or playing an instrument

☐ Discovering adult coloring books

☐ Enjoying the sensory pleasure of smell – a plant or flower

☐ Lighting candles all over, then sitting in the semi-darkness

☐ Having a spa night at home – bathing and grooming

☐ Savoring the sensory pleasure of taste – eating food slowly

☐ Curling up in a ball and listening to my favorite music

☐ Going for a swim or playing an evening sport

☐ Celebrating the sensory pleasure of touch – enjoying my skin

☐ Asking neighbors to come over and visit

☐ Learning something or taking up a new hobby

☐ Calling an old friend and catching up

☐ Writing three pages of Cycles by hand

☐ Playing classic games like checkers, cards, dominoes

☐ Making a community connection by telephone

☐ Making love or giving backrubs

☐ Sharing my hopes and dreams

☐ Reading to myself or aloud to my partner or child

Joy Dinner Ideas

☐ **Chicken and Veggie Salad**

A plate of fresh greens, topped with 6 oz. sliced chicken breast and 2 c. veggies, dressed with olive oil and balsamic vinegar.

☐ **Avocado and Shrimp Salad**

A plate of fresh greens, topped with one sliced avocado, ½ sliced cucumber, and 6 oz. cocktail shrimp, dressed with olive oil and sherry vinegar.

☐ **Turkey Breast, Artichoke, Greens, and Cherry Tomatoes**

Coat a turkey breast with olive oil and seasonings, bake, and slice. Meanwhile, cook an artichoke. Toss greens and cherry tomatoes in olive oil and vinegar. Arrange a plate of turkey, artichoke, and salad.

☐ **Teriyaki Chicken and Strawberry Pecan Salad**

Grill chicken breasts marinated in teriyaki sauce. Serve with salad greens topped with sliced strawberries and pecans, dressed with olive oil and balsamic vinegar.

☐ **Sautéed Snapper, Sliced Oranges, and Asparagus**

Sauté snapper or other fish in healthy oil, and top with sliced almonds, capers, and lemon juice. Serve with sliced oranges and steamed crisp asparagus.

☐ **Joe's Special Scramble**

Sauté ½ diced onion and ½ lb. ground round or ground turkey until the meat has browned and the onions are golden. Add 2 eggs, 2 c. leaf spinach, garlic, salt, and pepper to taste. Continue cooking until the eggs are firm and the spinach is wilted.

☐ **Freedom Salad**

Bed of greens of your choice, topped with 5 oz. of grilled wild-caught salmon, chicken breast, or flank steak, and your favorite veggies, dressed with olive oil, balsamic vinegar, and seasonings.

☐ **Nutty Chicken Salad**

Top a plate of fresh greens with a warm sliced chicken breast, and top with dried cranberries, sliced green onions, and walnut pieces. Drizzle with olive oil and vinegar.

☐ Turkey and Peppers

Shape ground turkey into ¼ lb. patties and season. Grill, then serve with sautéed red, green, and yellow peppers, and sliced tomatoes topped with olive oil.

☐ Pork Tenderloin, Avocado Salad, and Watermelon Wedges

Marinate pork tenderloin in hot mustard, vinaigrette, and peppers, then grill. Serve with sliced avocados and wedges of watermelon.

☐ London Broil Smothered in Mushrooms and Caesar Salad

Marinate meat in vinaigrette plus garlic and sweet hot mustard to taste. Sauté mushrooms in olive oil, broil steak, and serve with romaine, tomatoes, and cucumbers tossed with Caesar dressing.

☐ Quick Dinner Bowl

Sauté 2 c. of broccoli florets in extra virgin olive oil. Add leftover chicken, fish, or meat, and sauté until brown. Toast ½ c. nuts in frying pan on low heat until brown and fragrant. Season with favorite herbs, salt, and pepper. Combine ingredients and serve.

☐ Quick Vegan Bean Salad*^

Place dark greens (e.g., baby spinach and kale) on a plate. Heat up ¾ c. cooked beans of your choice in the microwave while slicing toppings of ½ avocado, ½ tomato, and ¼ chopped cucumber. Slide the beans onto the greens and add toppings. Drizzle with olive oil and vinegar. Add seasonings to taste.

☐ Fruit and Cottage Cheese Plate*

Slice up fruits that you love – cantaloupe, watermelon, peaches, bananas, kiwis, apples, oranges. Place a bed of lettuce on a plate and cover with 1 c. cottage cheese. Top with fruit and sprinkle with toasted wheat germ and sliced almonds.

☐ All Veggies and Nuts*^

Use a frying pan over medium to high heat and pour in 2 to 4 T. olive oil. Slice up onions, mushrooms, garlic, peppers, and other vegetables (e.g., cubed squash, yams, fennel, turnips, or carrots) and sauté each one separately, then combine them in the frying pan. Toast ¼ cup nuts in the frying pan until golden and add them with seasonings (e.g., salt, pepper, thyme, basil) and a splash of wine or broth and simmer for 5 minutes.

*contains agrarian foods
^not a high-protein meal

Success Check Day 20

- **Daily Success**

☐ I continued my Joy Practice with 10 Check Ins and 10 Joy Points.

☐ I reset my lifestyle in these seven ways: Exercise, Joy Breakfast, Sanctuary Time, Joy Lunch, Balancing Sleep, Natural Pleasure Binge, and Joy Dinner.

☐ I made one or more community connections for support with my lifestyle reset.

- **Did I pass the Success Check?   YES   NO**

If you did not, stay with this activity for one more day, then move on.

- **My Amazing Learning:**

_____

- **My Biggest Accomplishment:**

_____

- **My Biggest Challenge:**

_____

Beautiful Work!

You have completed Day 20 of The Joy Challenge.
Your next step is Day 21. Discover Your Body Circuit.

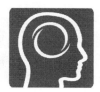

Day 21. Discover Your Body Circuit

Congratulations! You have developed your Power Grind Ins for Food, Mood, and Love. Now you are ready to clear the most important circuit of all: your Body Circuit. By clearing this wire, self-love will flow so strongly that releasing extra weight will be natural and a source of joy.

A Body Circuit is a ridiculous, rusty old wire that tells us to neglect or harm our body. Nearly everyone has one or two of these barbaric circuits, and crushing and transforming them is a very powerful act! Today we will discover that wire, so we can trounce it and reconfigure it in the days to come.

 A Body Circuit triggers us to neglect or harm our body.

When I began developing in 6th grade, a group of boys started making fun of me because of my weight. A wall went up inside me. My Body Circuit was encoded, and I started judging my body.

My older brother, Larry, was the jock in the family, and I was the uncoordinated skinny kid. The message from my family, particularly my dad, was that I needed to be big to be loved. My circuit of getting love from being big was encoded.

The Body Circuit

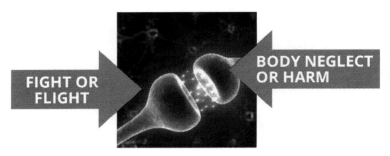

Two Types of Body Circuits

One type of Body Circuit tells us to judge our body, and the other tells us to use our body size for protection. These circuits are often encoded because we merge or distance, for example merging so that other people's ridiculous judgments of our body become encoded in our brain or distancing from someone by holding onto extra weight for protection.

Body Circuit Type 1: Body Judgment

The first type of Body Circuit is a judgment about our bodies. Perhaps someone criticizes our body, or we look at a model on a magazine cover and know we look nothing like that! The message worms its way into our unconscious mind and lodges itself there.

Why didn't we have boundaries to force it to go away? Usually, a Merge Circuit welcomes that Body Circuit of judgment. We merge with society and if the cultural norm is to look a certain way, we judge ourselves if that is not our look. We merge with parents, romantic partners, or friends who judge their bodies or our bodies and we "copy" their wire and start judging ourselves. Merging with them stops our nurturing inner voice from saying, "That is so ridiculous! Just because they judge me doesn't mean that I will judge myself!" The circuit settles into our brain.

Body Judgment Circuit

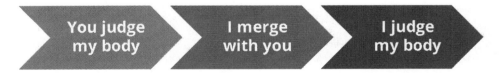

The Power Grind In for Love comes in handy when we rewire our Body Circuit of self-judgment. By using it, we can establish a healthy boundary. We have a healthy relationship with ourselves, stop the self-judgments, and love our body and ourselves. This is an extremely important boundary because there will always be people who make judgments and we give away our power and joy if we let their opinions take up residence in our brains.

Body Pride Circuit

| You judge my body | > | I do NOT merge with you | > | I love my body and myself |

Body Circuit Type 2: Self-Protection

The second type of Body Circuit is a bit more complex. This is a very deep circuit that is so central to survival that it is hidden in the furthest recesses of the unconscious mind. It is a circuit that tells us to manipulate our body size in order to meet our needs, such as safety, love, comfort, or pleasure.

The crossed wire between body size and protecting ourselves by meeting a basic need is completely illogical! However, it is extremely powerful and often the underlying cause of stress eating and weight issues.

One way of approaching this entire concept is to say to yourself, "My weight is perfect! It reflects the wires in my emotional brain. My body size is precisely what my emotional brain tells me is safe for me."

Emotional safety always trumps physical safety for us mammals, so if our emotional brain tells us to weigh a certain weight, then we will. What makes it safe to maintain a weight that is not actually a healthy weight? Almost any Stress Circuit can cause that. For that reason, our Advanced EBT Program focuses on clearing away all major Stress Circuits, as evidenced by having a high set point (wired at One). For example, a stressful experience that encodes the wire "I am bad" is soon generalized in the brain to I am always bad, and not only am I bad, but what I do is bad, and my body is bad. The experience of shame and being wrong, bad, or not enough is low in the brain and so threatening that it can encode a survival circuit that tells us to be at a body size that is "bad."

Also, traumatic experiences can encode a Food Circuit and overeating (or undereating) then leads to a change in weight. If we then experience that weight has given us safety, no matter how many logical people are telling us to change our weight, the reptile within will not let us, until we rewire that circuit!

When I was 10 years old, our neighbor, who was a good friend of our family, wanted me to sit on his lap. I was so innocent that I did it and he touched me inappropriately. I went numb and started binge eating after that. I never told anyone, but when I became heavy, it felt safe. Boys, and later men, stayed away from me. I didn't know how to use words to tell people to stay away from me and not to hit on me, but my body size expressed that for me. I was scared of being abused again and used my body size for protection.

If we do not get our safety from connecting to the deepest part of ourselves and being authentic, we encode circuits that attach us to various roles, such as I get my safety from being the super-achiever or the failure. In addition, we can encode survival circuits that give us a false sense of safety about who we are and easily become locked in and hard to change. For example, if our brain glitch is that we get our safety from being big, then anytime we lose weight, the reptile will have a fit and activate enough cortisol surges to make us overeat and regain the weight!

I have a jovial personality, and people think of me as a happy, big person. I think of my size as a big part of my identity. I am that big, friendly guy. I'm not sure people would like me if I lost weight. I have no skills to be close to others and that vulnerable, so I keep this extra layer of fat on my body to give me distance from them. Then I use this happy guy personality. I do not get the intimacy I need, which is stressful, so I eat more and cling even more to my large, happy guy body. I get my safety from my big, happy guy body.

We can use body size to give us an illusion of control over our own painful emotions. If we hold onto extra weight, perhaps we do not have to feel. It gives us some emotional armor, a layer of protection from our own emotional pain and from other people. Current relationships bring up circuits from past relationships that are full of unprocessed emotional pain, so even interacting with people who have a high set point and are objectively "safe" to be around can feel unsafe to us. It's that emotional trash that causes this.

In EBT, we use a combination of rewiring circuits and clearing away past hurts. Do not rush this process. Every Cycle you do to heal a hurt holds a nugget of truth in it, an awareness about the past that helps you know yourself in a new way. Healing is a process and leads to accessing more of the seven rewards of an exceptional life. The ongoing healing process is the source of our happiness.

I have a high-pressure job in a Fortune 500 company and I feel like an imposter because I am in way over my head. Every day I am frozen in fear that I am going to be found out and publicly humiliated. I live alone except for my two cats and even though I have broken my food wire and do not binge anymore, I still mindlessly eat.

I am not hungry, so I know there is a drive to hold onto extra weight. I know what that wire is. I get my survival from staying heavy. I can suppress my fears because I carry my own weight – literally. I distance from my co-workers and from myself by having this extra padding.

Self-Protection Circuit

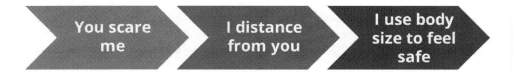

Body size is so meaningful that we unconsciously use it to express ourselves in a myriad of ways when we distance from others to not feel our feelings or express our needs. The ways this shows up are endless. Here are a few common examples:

I started dating Carl and he was about 20 pounds overweight and had just had a heart attack. We were in the falling-in-love stage and you could blame my 15-pound weight gain on eating chocolate, but in truth, it was a Body Circuit of showing my solidarity with him. I was merged enough that I would do anything for his approval and distanced enough that I didn't use words to tell him that I worried about his weight because of his health. Instead, I joined him by gaining weight. I get my security from being as fat as he is.

Body Pride Circuit

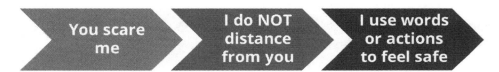

I keep about 10 pounds of extra weight around my thighs and never realized it was perfect. My body circuit was telling me to hold onto that weight. I have a sister who is going through a divorce and a brother who is an alcoholic and I don't have any problems – I have a happy marriage, two great kids, and a job I love – and I don't know how to talk about what's going on in my life and theirs with my siblings. I hold onto 10 extra pounds as my ridiculous way of not superseding them or feeling like I am better than them. I get my love from packing around 10 extra pounds.

I am not overweight or underweight. My weight and my body are as perfect as I can make them. I have that "body perfect" syndrome and it is not out of body pride. I obsess about my appearance which is what everyone calls me on. They tell me that I am addicted to my looks, but they have no idea that I am an anxious wreck. I'm constantly miserable. I have an Anxiety Circuit that is as thick as a tree trunk! I don't share how I feel. My Body Circuit protects me because I can get my false sense of security by having my body be absolutely and completely perfect.

The seesaw of merging and distancing plays into family obesity too, or even a family need to manipulate weight, weight cycle, or talk about weight, rather than other deeper matters that could bring intimacy and connection. There are lots of family circuits being activated, but one of them is the Body Circuit.

Everyone in our family loves to eat and expresses their love for each other with food. We are all 20 to 40 pounds overweight. It's a family tradition. I know it's not genetic because my younger sister looks just like me. She somehow escaped the Body Circuit of our family. Of course, we NEVER talk about it, but after doing a dozen or so Cycles about it, I found my Body Circuit. It is I get my protection of family love from being precisely as heavy as they are. For short it is: I get my security from a body that is like my family's bodies. That is a merge! It's also a distancing circuit. Our entire family has diabetes and nobody is talking about how we eat or what we weigh! My first step: transform my Body Circuit.

With our Power Grind In for Love handy, short-circuiting merging and distancing, we can create a healthy boundary about our body. This is essential. We cannot merge with people and use body size to protect ourselves. We cannot let other people's inane judgments of our body reach us.

When I fried this circuit, I fell in love with my body and myself. Eating healthy and being slightly hungry were nurturing acts. I wanted my outside to reflect the person I was inside. Releasing weight was natural.

Why

We rewire this circuit because it effectively blocks our drive to eat healthy and release extra weight. This circuit may be the most important of the four wires for ending overeating. The unconscious mind is very powerful and if our emotional brain is telling us to hold onto extra weight to be safe, then we will do that no matter what. If our emotional brain is giving us strong messages that our body is bad, we will neglect or abuse our body. By frying this circuit, healthy eating becomes sensible and fun and the extra weight either slowly departs or we shed it quickly. It's not consistent with who we are anymore.

How

We rewire this circuit just like we rewired the first three. Complain that you cannot lose weight. Complain that you do not like your body. Complain about regaining weight. All you must do is complain and the Cycle Tool will process that complaint and take you right to your Body Circuit!

The situation is . . . I hate my body. It has a big stomach and huge thighs and breasts that have a mind of their own and I carry this body with me every day. It is a bad body and I don't know what to do about it. What I'm most stressed about is . . . I have a bad body. I feel ANGRY I have this body. I can't stand it that I have this body. I HATE HATE HATE my body!!! . . . My mind went blank. I unlocked the circuit . . . I feel sad that . . . I have this body. I feel afraid that . . . nobody will love this body. I feel guilty that . . . I don't love my body. OF COURSE I don't love my body, because I get my . . . safety from hating my body and myself. That's really gross! I have a wire that tells me to hate my body and myself. My whole body is tingling. I found my Body Circuit!

The situation is . . . I started gaining weight when my parents divorced. I was nine years old and I would steal food from the cupboards and stuff myself with candy. I gained weight and my father was so hard on me about it. I was meek and never told him how much I hated his judgments, except that I just kept eating. I kept getting bigger and he got even more frustrated with me. What I'm most stressed about is . . . I am 34 years old and I am very overweight. I feel angry that I am overweight. I can't stand it that I did this to myself. I HATE it that I don't give a &#%$ about my body. I HATE IT that I don't care about my health. I HATE it that I keep on all this weight. I HATE IT! . . . which makes me sad. I feel sad that . . . I weigh so much. I feel afraid that . . . I am going to destroy my health. I feel guilty that . . . I hold onto this weight. It must be an old wire. OF COURSE I hold onto this weight, because my unreasonable expectation is . . . I get my power from being fat. I get my existence from being fat. I get my need to rebel against my father from being fat. I get my everything from being fat. Okay, take a deep breath. OF COURSE I hold onto my weight, because I get my existence from being big. That's the one. I get my existence from being big!

Body Circuit Examples

Type	Examples
Body Judgment	• I get my safety from judging my body. • I get my comfort from telling myself I am unattractive. • I get my survival from having disgust for my body. • I get my power from hating my body. • I get my pleasure from ridiculing my body. • I get my love from being critical of my appearance.
Self-Protection	• I get my safety from being big. • I get my existence from being invisible. • I get my love from losing and gaining weight. • I get my security from using body size as body armor. • I get my comfort from carrying around extra weight. • I get my protection from neglecting my body.

Seeing the circuit, grieving the circuit, and traveling back

You have already discovered three circuits and know how to warmly observe a circuit, feel your feelings about it, travel back on it, and more. However, for this wire, please take extra time to make friends with it, to be aware that it has been sitting in your brain for some time, and to love that wire. It was only encoded to protect you, because given the environment you lived in, your situational stress, and your merging or distancing circuits, that was the best your brain could do.

Feel tenderly toward that circuit and prepare for tomorrow's activity. You will unravel that wire, so you have more freedom to love your body, and, in time, to notice a growing desire to release extra weight. When you stop needing extra weight because you've trained your brain for unconditional love and intense joy, then releasing it becomes natural, pleasurable, and surprisingly easy. Prior to that, releasing weight feels either impossible or like agony.

My size felt good to me. Then my set point changed, or something changed, and I wanted to get out of that body. It wasn't "me" anymore.

When my body pride switch turned on, my rebellion against my parents, men, society, and corporations stopped. I didn't care about them. I wanted my healthy body size back.

As your brain changes, your life changes in radical ways. Your need is not for the weight or the food. Your need is for the freedom to reclaim your genetic body build. It is to enjoy your body in its perfectly imperfect state! You can experience this! That is the power of the brain to change your mindset and your experience of life.

The Rewiring Checklist
Day 1. Discover Your Body Circuit

Say What Is Bothering You

- The situation is . . . (Complain about your body.)
- What I'm most stressed about is . . . (Say what bothers you most about your body.)

Unlock the Circuit

- I feel angry that . . .
- I can't stand it that . . .
- I hate it that . . .

Discover the Hidden Message

- I feel sad that . . .
- I feel afraid that . . .
- I feel guilty that . . .
- OF COURSE I would do that, because my unreasonable expectation is . . .

I get my:	from:	
	BODY JUDGMENT	**SELF-PROTECTION**
☐ Safety		
☐ Love	☐ Doubting my attractiveness	☐ Staying heavy
☐ Comfort	☐ Rejecting my body	☐ Being big
☐ Pleasure	☐ Feeling disgust for my body	☐ Carrying extra pounds
☐ Purpose	☐ Hating my body	☐ Being underweight
☐ Survival	☐ Ridiculing my body	☐ Using size as body armor
☐ Existence	☐ Being critical of my body	☐ Gaining and losing weight
☐ Protection	☐ Finding fault with my body	☐ Being invisible
☐ Security	☐ Demanding body perfection	☐ Neglecting my body
☐ Power	☐ Obsessing on body problems	☐ Using my body as protection
☐ Nurturing	☐ Disliking my body	☐ Abusing my body
☐ Other _____	☐ Other _____	☐ Other _____

Success Check Day 21

- **Daily Success**

  ☐ I continued my Joy Practice with 10 Check Ins and 10 Joy Points.

  ☐ I discovered my Body Circuit.

  ☐ I made one or more community connections for support with discovering my circuit.

- **Did I pass the Success Check?   YES   NO**

  If you did not, stay with this activity for one more day, then move on.

- **My Amazing Learning:**

  _____

- **My Biggest Accomplishment:**

  _____

- **My Biggest Challenge:**

  _____

Congratulations!

**You have completed Day 21 of The Joy Challenge.
Your next step is Day 22. Negate Your Body Circuit.**

Day 22. Negate Your Body Circuit

Today we will negate our Body Circuit. This is a great day! You are doing something that will bring you freedom and joy.

You might need to take out more emotional trash. Be liberal with Cycles, doing five of them, then another five, even more. It hurts to have a Body Circuit. It takes as long as it takes to grieve it! Cycle on this until you have a zest for crushing this circuit!

We are vivid emotional and spiritual beings, but our only irreplaceable possession is our body. We must crush that circuit which encoded itself without our permission or awareness. Instead of letting that circuit turn us against ourselves, we will transform it into a wire that deepens our love, respect, and caring for ourselves.

Today we will negate that circuit, rip it apart, and make sure that it will no longer control our weight or shut down our natural drive to love our bodies. This will activate the joy of releasing extra weight.

Why

When the Body Circuit transforms into a wire that supports our body pride, a cascade of changes follows. When I was in my mid-20s, I worked for a woman who had body pride. She loved her body, celebrated her sensuality, and saw her body as another gift of life – something she enjoyed. Body pride was a new concept for me.

One day she passed by my desk and said, "Laurel, why don't you have fun with your body? Why don't you play with it and celebrate it?"

At the time, I had no words to respond to her. I had not heard about the "fun" part of having a body before, and I didn't know that it was an old circuit of body shame that blocked my pride. Nor did I understand the joy of releasing extra weight.

When we connect with ourselves so deeply and really like and love ourselves, we create a self-nurturing boundary. We are not going to look the way other people want us to look. We are not going to rebel against the judgments of others. All that matters is that we love our body and take really good care of it. If our weight is above our genetic body build, the padding seems extra. The love we show ourselves inside begs to be expressed by our love for our flesh and blood, and our body shape and size. Instead of needing the extra weight for safety, love, comfort, or pleasure, we can't wait to be FREE of that weight.

Until we have that excitement about coming out of our old body – unzipping it and stepping out of it – into a new body, then it will not be fun to release extra weight. And if it's not fun, it's not EBT. By crushing this circuit, that desire to release extra weight, celebrate, and have fun with our body takes over. When you least expect it, something deep within you will shift! You will not need that weight anymore. You cherish yourself in a new way and want to release the extra weight.

I'm so glad I broke my Body Circuit. Words started tumbling out of my mouth that I never imagined I would say. An entirely new attitude toward food suddenly appeared. Hunger? Great! That's a sign that I'm releasing weight! Eat kale and broccoli? How delicious!

How

Use the same negation process you used with your Food and Mood Circuits. First, stress-activate the wire by stating the unreasonable expectation, such as, "I get my safety from neglecting my body." Or, watch for moments when the circuit is activated by daily stress. Pause for one to 10 minutes until you are at Brain State 3, then negate the circuit slowly, then ridicule it. Have fun dismantling that ridiculous circuit!

2 Stages of Negating a Body Circuit	
SLOW	I . . . can . . . NOT . . . get . . . my . . . power . . . from . . . ignoring my body. I . . . can . . . NOT . . . get . . . my . . . power . . . from . . . ignoring my body. I . . . can . . . NOT . . . get . . . my . . . power . . . from . . . ignoring my body. I . . . can . . . NOT . . . get . . . my . . . power . . . from . . . ignoring my body.
RAMP UP	That's ridiculous! I can NOT get power from IGNORING my body. Forget that! Ignoring my body is sad and silly. It does NOT give me power. Ignoring my body is harmful. I can NOT get power from doing something that ridiculous! I CANNOT get POWER from IGNORING my body! NEVER COULD. NEVER WILL.

Example (All Grind In Clusters count as 10 Grind Ins)

SLOW

- I . . . can . . . NOT . . . get . . . SAFETY . . . from . . . staying heavy . . . (pause)
- I . . . can . . . NOT . . . get . . . SAFETY . . . from . . . staying heavy . . . (pause)
- I . . . can . . . NOT . . . get . . . SAFETY . . . from . . . staying heavy . . . (pause)
- I . . . can . . . NOT . . . get . . . SAFETY . . . from . . . staying heavy . . . (pause)
- I . . . can . . . NOT . . . get . . . SAFETY . . . from . . . staying heavy . . . (pause)

RAMP UP

- That's ridiculous! I can NOT get safety from staying heavy.
- Staying heavy does NOT make me safe.
- Carrying around extra weight does NOT give me the safety that I need.
- That's ridiculous! I CANNOT get safety from holding onto extra weight!
- Totally RIDICULOUS! I can NOT get safety from staying heavy.
- I CANNOT GET MY SAFETY from STAYING HEAVY!!!

If it's not fun, do 5 Cycles, then negate the wire

Be sure to grieve. Think of the grieving like this: The moment when your unconscious mind registered that judging your body or holding onto extra weight made you safe, things were not going well. You were not surrounded by love, warmth, kindness, and people who had reasonable expectations and could share their wisdom with you. That alone is worth grieving!

As well, you have made decisions about eating and weight that were controlled by the primitive and powerful unconscious mind. These are survival circuits and we had no way of knowing they are calling the shots when it came to our eating and weight – until now. You have been blindsided, so it makes sense that you would grieve your losses. You have been hurt. Feeling the feelings by cycling about this is healing. Take your time to grieve!

The situation is . . . I have been overweight since age five. I do get my safety from holding onto weight, because that's what my parents did. They held onto their weight, and I didn't know how to do anything but hold onto my weight. I would be lost if I did not have my weight. It does comfort me. What I'm most stressed about is . . . I hold onto weight. I feel ANGRY that a stupid wire tells me to hold onto my weight. I can't stand it that this wire has ordered me around. I HATE it that I have believed this wire. I HATE THAT!!!! . . . I really REALLY HATE that!!! . . . which makes me sad. I feel sad that . . . I believed this circuit . . . I feel afraid that . . . I will not know what to do without it . . . I am afraid I will be lost if I do not get my safety from these extra pounds. I feel guilty that . . . I didn't know it was a wire. OF COURSE I would feel guilty that I didn't know it was a wire, because my unreasonable expectation is . . . I should figure everything out and never let anything or anyone delude me. That's it. I have to be perfectly wise all the time. I do NOT have to be perfectly wise all the time. That's ridiculous! Nobody is perfectly wise all the time. All I have to do is keep learning, changing, growing, and becoming

- Sing your Grind In while showering or bathing.
- Use it while you dress or undress.
- State your Grind In while stroking your body.
- Say it as you clean out your closet to update your look.
- Say your Grind In with fury as you view "body perfect" magazines.

wiser and wiser, and more and more joyful day by day! All I need to do is give myself unconditional love no matter what! All I have to do is connect to the deepest part of myself and love myself, truly and profoundly love myself! I can do that. I am going to do that!

Let's stomp that circuit with Power Boosters

Enjoy your power to train your brain. Right now, your Grind In is a way for your neocortex to deliver experiences to your unconscious mind. The more you confront this circuit with passion and repetition, contradicting the old message, the more the unconscious message changes.

It's our unconscious messages that we obey when it comes to anything primitive and fundamental, like accessing safety by judging our body or holding onto extra weight. When we break the faulty circuit, we feel the difference. We relax! We unleash a natural drive to lose weight and eat healthy.

My Body Circuit was encoded when my mother shamed me for being too fat. Some rage came up in me, and my brain encoded a wire to get my safety by getting back at her and being as fat as I could be. After a few years, I was comfortable with my size. In fact, I wasn't even sure if anyone would like me if I were not fat. It went with my personality of being the round and nice person who everyone likes. When I broke that wire, I noticed that my big body was not right for me anymore. I was well on my way to rewiring my merging circuit and I wasn't willing to be heavy in order for people to like me. Also, I had expressed my rage about my mother's judgments of my body. I must have done 20 Cycles on my mother, but I did one more Cycle and the stress lifted. I started losing weight, and for the first time in my life, it was not hard at all. The problem all along was not me. It was a faulty circuit.

The solution is to train your brain, and when you "feel the difference," you know that you have broken that circuit! When you spontaneously love your body and feel excited about releasing weight, you have crushed the old wire. That is not only fun and exciting, but it starts a new chapter in our lives!

 Holding onto weight will not give me the safety I need.

The Rewiring Checklist
Day 2. Negate Your Body Circuit

I activated my Body Circuit by stating my unreasonable expectation, then paused until I was at Brain State 3. Then I negated it:

- **SLOW**

    I can NOT get my _____ from _____.

- **RAMP UP**

    That's ridiculous! I can NOT get my _____ from _____.

    I negated it: 50   75   100   125   150   200 _____ times.

I boosted the power of my Grind In (one or more ways):

☐   Singing my Grind In while showering or bathing

☐   Using it while I dress or undress

☐   Stating my Grind In while stroking my body

☐   Saying it as I clean out my closets to update my look

☐   Saying my Grind In with fury as I view "body perfect" magazines

Success Check Day 22

● **Daily Success**

☐ I continued my Joy Practice with 10 Check Ins and 10 Joy Points.

☐ I negated my Body Circuit.

☐ I made one or more community connections for support with negating my circuit.

● **Did I pass the Success Check?   YES   NO**

If you did not, stay with this activity for one more day, then move on.

● **My Amazing Learning:**

_____

● **My Biggest Accomplishment:**

_____

● **My Biggest Challenge:**

_____

Great Work!

You have completed Day 22 of The Joy Challenge.
Your next step is Day 23. Transform Your Body Circuit.

Day 23. Transform Your Body Circuit

Of all the circuits you will ever rewire, this one may be the most important. Today you will create a Power Grind In for your Body Circuit.

This Power Grind In will act as a protective shield, you feel love – unconditional love – for yourself and your body. Releasing weight becomes natural, in fact, a joy.

I want my body to show who I really am, a person who loves herself and her body. These handfuls of extra weight? I'm releasing them.

Natural, Lasting Weight Loss

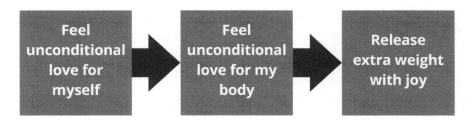

Why

Fundamental to our survival is that we have wires in our unconscious mind that encode a drive to love our body and take care of our body. If we have wires that have been encoded by our experiences that cause us to judge our body, neglect our body, abuse our body, or not protect our body, they must be cleared if we are to be healthy and happy. Until we have rearranged our relationship with our body, why would we go to the effort to have body pride, eat for vibrancy or freedom, and be at peace with ourselves? You have already developed Power Grind Ins to rewire three other circuits. This fourth circuit is often the deepest, most sensitive one, and when we clear it, we reset our brain to fall in love not only with our body but with ourself!

I have my mother's body-hatred in my emotional brain. Now I'm passing that along to my daughter who is already judging her body as if she were an object. I am furious that I have that circuit, and I'm going to fry it!

How
Create your Power Grind In for your body with precision. Install in your brain a new message that will be life-changing. Use three parts to the new message: the three-pronged transformation.

Connect: Tell yourself to connect within, in whatever way sounds right to you. You may have one connect statement you like best, that you use for all Power Grind Ins, or you may vary them. Whatever feels really good to say will work the best.

Approach: State how you are going to replace judging your body or protecting yourself by maintaining a body size that is not consistent with your genetic body build. What will be your new approach to your body?

Reward: What is the reward that makes staying present and aware worth the effort? Is it Sanctuary, Authenticity, Vibrancy, Integrity, Intimacy, Spirituality, or Freedom?

Where is your circuit stored?
As with the other circuits, this wire was encoded because you had an unmet need. Your brain had no wire to help you meet that need, and it was so overwhelmed in the moment that it created a false association between that need and either body shame or holding onto extra weight.

Most Body Circuits for self-protection are stored in the 5th Drawer of the brain. It's the 5th Drawer that stores our survival circuits. These circuits are perceived by the brain as so core to sustaining our existence that our mind goes blank when we try to activate them. We hold onto the weight because our reptilian brain shuts down our capacity to clear away that wire!

Self-judgment wires can be stored in any of the drawers, from mild annoyance at our body to outright hatred toward it. Your conscious mind did not encode this circuit but ONLY your conscious mind breaking this wire can change it. Use all the power you need to crush that circuit. Determine where it is stored in order to construct an effective plan.

Select your approach to your body
Select a new relationship with your body. You have the power to do that. Use your power in a truly responsive way. Choose among these approaches:

The Body Love Approach
Decide to reject any trace of body judgment that has crept into your brain in the past and become lodged there as well as any new influx of body judgment from a world that treats people like objects and has yet to evolve and be powered by compassion, love, and joy. With this approach, you have the option to change your body, but that change is rooted in one thing: self-love.

This extra weight is a sign that I did not have the skills to comfort myself from within, so I needed the food. So what? That was my need and I will never judge myself for that, nor will I ever judge the size of my body. No Judgments! NONE!

I am very short (5'1") and grew up in a family of tall people. My dad gave me direct messages that I was less because I was short. I became an overachiever and moved up the ladder in my company quickly, but the more my career progressed, the more anxious I became. I put on 50 pounds because my wire was that I get my power from being big. I hate that I did not have a wire to get my safety from inside of me and find love for my perfect and short body. I'm going to encode that wire for myself!

I wish I had these tools 20 years ago and had loved my body then. I neglected my body and my skin looks so old. How perfect. My body is telling me to connect with myself and my body and to start being kinder to myself and taking really good care of myself out of pure LOVE!

Body Love Approach Examples
• **Love my body unconditionally.** • **Celebrate my BODY PRIDE!** • **Feel love for my body and myself.** • **Release extra weight out of self-love.** • **Stop JUDGING my body. LOVE my body!**

The Be Strong and Healthy Approach

Imagine your hunter-gatherer ancestors. They needed their body to be sturdy because there was no plethora of medications, procedures, and devices to prop them up. They had to be healthy from the inside out, with a lifestyle that made their brain and body strong. We become weaker as individuals and as a society by skipping healthy living in favor of dependency on drugs. No drugs can replace healthy living!

My approach to my body is to get back to basics and be as healthy and strong as I can be. I have no room for judgments and I will not carry extra weight. I want to live clean and treat my body with love and respect.

Food was love for me. I always cleaned my plate to please my mom. Also, it was a toy, a source of pleasure and fun. There was no association between eating healthy and keeping a healthy weight in my family. My approach is to make my body strong, so I feel great! My rewards? Vibrancy . . . and Integrity.

Be Strong and Healthy Approach Examples

- Be at a weight that makes me vibrant!
- Make my body strong and healthy.
- Take excellent care of my body.
- Be healthy with a zest for life.
- Reclaim my genetic body build!

The Meet My Need Approach

Bring to mind why your brain encoded this circuit. You had an unmet need. Your approach statement directs you to meet that need. By taking extra care to build into your life ways you will meet that need, your natural drive for body pride will emerge.

I encoded my Food Circuit when my first husband disappeared one day, leaving me with a toddler and a slew of unpaid bills. I ate my way through that, but never really appreciated that I had no idea how to comfort myself in healthy ways. I am going to encode that I stay reasonably connected to myself and comfort myself in healthy ways. My reward? Intimacy. That's not logical, but that's what bubbled up from my body and rings true to me. That's my new circuit!

My Body Circuit was encoded right after a violent incident in our home that changed things for my whole family. I was fortunate in that I had a lot of counseling right away and kept that trauma (survival) circuit from settling into my brain, but a sense of comfort never returned for me. To this day I do not know how to comfort myself other than staying chubby or eating and drinking. I want to deal with that skill deficit and encode a wire of soothing and comforting myself in healthy ways.

Meet My Need Approach Examples

- Meet my true need, rather than judging my body.
- Get my safety from inside me, not from staying big.
- Get my love from inside me, not from carrying extra weight.
- Comfort myself in healthy ways.
- Feast on natural pleasures.
- Bring my mind my reward for body pride.

The Body Circuit Imagine

Use this Imagine to fine-tune your transformation statement for your Power Grind In for your Body Circuit. Have fun with it!

Relax: Find a place that is private and get comfortable. Focus your attention on your body and your breathing in any way that is comforting and comfortable to you. When you are ready, begin to imagine.

Imagine: See yourself awakening in the morning and taking a few moments to experience body pride. It might mean rolling over in bed and noticing the feel of your skin on the sheets or curling up in a ball, hugging your own body. Start your day stating that you are creating joy in your life, then imagine yourself moving through your day doing just that.

Next, see yourself activating your circuits of body pride and enjoying feeling connected to your body, aware of your sensations and emotions, and feeling loving toward your body and yourself. However, that Body Circuit is still rumbling around in the very bottom of your brain and you sense that.

See yourself moving into a stressful time of the day, just the situation in which your Body Circuit could be activated.

See yourself pulling out your Power Grind In for Body and short-circuiting that wire. It's a beautiful experience because you are saying to yourself the words that you most need to hear, the words that, if you had heard them early in life, would have blocked that Body Circuit from ever being encoded.

Use the precise words you need to hear to instruct yourself to connect with yourself . . . words that are clear and supportive . . . Then state your new approach to your body . . . Use words that tell you precisely how to approach this challenge to your body pride.

Last, consider which reward will motivate you to short-circuit that wire and replace it with a new body pride circuit . . . whether it is . . . Sanctuary, Authenticity, Vibrancy, Integrity, Intimacy, Spirituality, or Freedom.

Please take all the time you need. Then use the upcoming checklist to record the transformation statement that feels right to you.

The Power Grind In for Body:
Protection Example

Stage	Statements
1 SLOW	I can NOT get my love from rejecting my body.
2 RAMP UP	That's ridiculous! I can NOT get the love I need from rejecting my body. How mean that is! That's ridiculous. I can NOT get love from rejecting my precious body. That's absolutely crazy!
3 JOY	I get love from connecting to myself and loving my body, imperfections and all. Reward: Vibrancy. I get love from connecting to MYSELF and giving my body unconditional love. Reward: It's Vibrancy. I GET LOVE from connecting to myself and loving my body! Reward: Vibrancy . . . feeling healthy with a ZEST for life!

For many people, this Body Circuit is the "missing link" in ending overeating and creating lasting weight loss. Take all the time you need to discover the words that feel right to you. Once you have created this Grind In, you will have a secure base with each of your four Power Grind Ins. Continue with a lifestyle reset for body pride and then move right on to jumpstarting raising your set point.

The Power Grind In for Body:
Judgment Example

Stage	Statements
1 SLOW	I can NOT get my safety from extra weight.
2 RAMP UP	Carrying around extra weight is NOT going to give me the safety I need. How ridiculous! I can NOT get safety from extra weight. Completely ridiculous!
3 JOY	I get my safety from connecting to the power inside me, and releasing this extra weight. Reward: Freedom. I get my safety from connecting to the power inside me, and releasing this extra weight. Reward: FREEDOM. I get MY SAFETY from connecting to the power inside me, and releasing this extra weight. Reward: FREEDOM!!!

As you transition from establishing your four Power Grind Ins, the reptile could be very snappish. Keep your sense of humor, and when your success in raising your set point is significant enough to cause a Brain State 5, use the tools and appreciate your success.

Create your Power Grind In for Body

Develop your Power Grind In for Body. Experiment until you find the words that are right for you. Make solid a new approach to your body, a new relationship with your physical presence on this planet.

Creating the right Power Grind In took time. I was second-guessing myself about which circuit I would rewire. Then I realized that the one I put on the shelf for now was not going to go anywhere. It would still be there when I got around to rewiring it. Or, if it was gone because another rewiring swept it away, I'd know it. I'm learning to let go of being in complete control of my emotional wires all the time!

The Rewiring Checklist
Day 3. Transform Your Body Circuit

After activating my Body Circuit by stating my unreasonable expectation, I paused until I was at Brain State 3. Then I transformed it:

- **SLOW**

  I can NOT get my _____ from _____.

- **RAMP UP**

  That's ridiculous! I can NOT get my _____ from _____.

- **JOY**

I get my: _____ **from:**

CONNECT	APPROACH	REWARD
☐ Connecting with myself	☐ Releasing weight for a purpose	☐ Sanctuary
☐ Checking in	☐ Reclaiming my genetic body build	☐ Authenticity
☐ Knowing my number	☐ Choosing healthy comforts	☐ Vibrancy
☐ Honoring my feelings	☐ STOP hating my body and myself!	☐ Integrity
☐ Loving myself	☐ Creating safety from within	☐ Intimacy
☐ The compassion within	☐ Loving my body unconditionally	☐ Spirituality
☐ Honoring my strengths	☐ Taking excellent care of my body	☐ Freedom
☐ Believing in myself	☐ Releasing extra weight out of self-love	
☐ Trusting myself	☐ LOVING my body, no more JUDGING it	
☐ Listening to my body	☐ NEVER judging my body, no matter what!	
☐ Being present now	☐ Celebrating MY BODY PRIDE!	
☐ Other _____	☐ Other _____	

I transformed it: 50   75   100   125   150   200 _____ times.

Success Check Day 23

- **Daily Success**

☐ I continued my Joy Practice with 10 Check Ins and 10 Joy Points.

☐ I transformed my Body Circuit and created my Power Grind In.

☐ I made one or more community connections for support with transforming my circuit.

- **Did I pass the Success Check?   YES   NO**

If you did not, stay with this activity for one more day, then move on.

- **My Amazing Learning:**

_____

- **My Biggest Accomplishment:**

_____

- **My Biggest Challenge:**

_____

Beautiful Work!

You have completed Day 23 of The Joy Challenge.
Your next step is Day 24. Lifestyle Reset #5
Body Pride and Sensual Pleasure.

Day 24. Lifestyle Reset #5
Body Pride and Sensual Pleasure

You've changed so much on the inside, it's time to reset your relationship with your body and the natural pleasures of life in two areas. One is body pride, enjoying your body, and the other is sensual pleasure, amplifying the sensory rewards you experience at Brain State 1.

- **Reset your connection with your body.**
- **Enjoy a new level of body pride.**
- **Celebrate your sensual nature.**

Why

As your set point rises, you will continue to experience your body in a new way. Stress causes us to disconnect from our body and treat our body like an object. We become self-critical, judgmental, dismissive, or detached, and stop short of enjoying the sensory pleasure inherent to our physical nature. The state of connection to our body becomes more apparent as we spend more moments of the day at One.

I was dressing for work this morning and these words bubbled up to my consciousness: "You look good, Dear." I was shocked. When have I ever spoken to myself with such kindness – and been so accepting of my body? Never!

My best Joy Points are from sensory pleasures, but I have recently extended that to being more sensual. My stress mode is to overthink and to be an introvert. In the past, I was always so immersed in my neocortex. Lately, I have been enjoying using my senses to make me happy. I was driving my six-year-old son to school and I told him to look out the window and name three colors he saw in the clouds. I never would have done that a month ago!

Body Pride
Knowing, honoring, and celebrating your appearance

Sensual Pleasure
Enjoying your body's senses, appetites, and passions

All bodies are perfect bodies

As our set point continues to rise, the hypercritical reptile voice about our bodies seems so frighteningly immature. In its place comes not only a desire to take really good care of our bodies, adorn them, and celebrate them, but a great deal of respect and appreciation for our physical presence on the planet.

My body shows my personal history. After I found out about my husband's affair with a co-worker, my set point went to 4.5. I did not have the emotional skills to process the betrayal. I did exactly what I needed to do at the time: eat and drink my way through the pain. I hated how I looked: puffy and big. I did a deep Cycle and realized that my body was perfect in its own way. My body showed what I had been through. Accepting that this happened, and that my body showed the hurt, made me calm. I was energized to get healthy, take care of my body, and begin again.

I was in the store looking for tops with long sleeves and couldn't find many. I complained to the salesperson. I said, "The skin on my arms is starting to sag. I need to cover them up." She looked back at me and said, "Well, at least you have arms. Perhaps you should celebrate that!" I bought a sleeveless dress. Away went body shame and I switched over to body pride. All bodies are good bodies, including mine.

Why oxytocin matters!

Oxytocin is the empathy hormone
which is stimulated by emotional connection.
It is a powerful appetite suppressant.

"I lovingly connect with people – and eat less."

Clear away that emotional clutter!

To reset your relationship with your body, bringing your "outside" body in line with your emotional and spiritual core, requires clearing away some emotional clutter. This is true for everyone and, going forward, it will be part of your EBT practice. Any insult or odd expectation that happens to drop into your emotional brain, you clear it away. Think of it as daily emotional cleansing!

Right now, let's do some "spring cleaning" and clear away some clutter that accumulated in the pre-EBT days. Do a few Cycles and notice a fresh attitude toward your body and yourself.

The situation is . . . I love my body, and I am excited about this reset. Today I'll savor sensual pleasure, but not so much that my reptilian brain hisses at me. What I'm most stressed about is . . . I have denied myself "body fun" for so long. I feel angry that I have denied myself this pleasure. I can't stand it that I had a free source of joy and didn't use it. I HATE IT that I can't get that time back! . . . I feel sad . . . that I lost that time. I feel afraid that . . . I can't play with my body now. I feel guilty that . . . I am so scared about playing with my own body! Of course I'm scared about playing with my body, because my unreasonable expectation is . . . I get my safety from denying myself pleasure. Oh, wow, that's fascinating. No wonder I used to need food so much and used to shut down body pleasures. I can NOT get my safety from denying myself pleasure. I can NOT get my safety from denying myself pleasure. That's ridiculous. Denying myself pleasure is NO WAY to give me safety. It just makes me crave artificial rewards. I get my safety from connecting to myself, enjoying the rich pleasures of my life. My reward? Vibrancy!

The situation is . . . my pants are loose and putting on old clothes that I used to hide in feels . . . out of authenticity. I'm not that person anymore. What I'm most stressed about is . . . I am not a fat person anymore, but my mind thinks I am. No, that's not it. I am leaving my fat body for a new body size. I feel angry that . . . I am mixed up about my body (Maybe I'm at 5). I can't stand it that . . . my body is changing. I HATE it that I do not know who I am anymore. I HATE it that I am confused! I HATE THAT!!! I really HATE that!!! . . . I feel sad that . . . I am changing. . . I feel afraid that . . . I am going to freak out and go back to my old body . . . I feel guilty that . . . I am so stressed about all this . . . Of course I am stressed about this, because my unreasonable expectation is that I must feel secure all the time. I get my safety from feeling secure all the time. That's ridiculous. I cannot get my safety from feeling secure all the time. I get my safety from connecting with the safe place inside me, processing my wild and woolly emotions, and living a full, dynamic, and ever-changing life! My reward? Sanctuary.

Enjoying sensual pleasure

Stress shuts down sensory awareness and distorts the sensual nature of life. The four most common sexual issues in men and women are caused by stress. If we are stressed, the first thing to go is sex drive (arousal and desire).

The emotional brain is the #1 sex organ, so as our set point rises, often we renew our awareness first of our senses, then of the sensual pleasures of life. Our sexuality is core to our sense of self and loving connection. Sensual pleasures also increase oxytocin, which is a powerful appetite suppressant!

I am enjoying all my senses more, particularly touch. When I can't sleep at night, I run my hands over my skin and notice how it feels. I have bumps on my skin and I feel them. I run my fingertips down my arms. It sounds like an inconsequential thing, but I didn't do that in the past.

After we had children, my wife and I distanced from each other. After dinner, she would go into the kitchen to eat and I would go to my computer to work and fume. Last night we made love. Somehow she overcame her low desire and I stopped fuming and started feeling more love for her. Our brains are changing!

Celebrate your body!

Celebrate your amazing body. Your body reflects your personal history and life journey, which always has a good side to it. If your body shows what you have been through, celebrate all the good that came from those experiences. Mourn the losses, then love your body, celebrate your body, and have fun with your body!

I have stretch marks on my legs and breasts from pregnancies. The light side is that I have two children. I'm going to be happy I have my kids and see those marks as an accomplishment. I am living life as a mother and that's what I want to do! I will model for my two daughters that they do not have to have a perfect body to have a beautiful body! What a wonderful opportunity to share healthy wires with them.

I was complaining about my body to my wife and she said, "I'm sorry that you do not have body pride. How can I help?" I did some Cycles and found the power to love my body unconditionally. I started eating less. It's not logical but that is what happened for me.

How

See how many of the strategies listed on the following two pages you will try out to give yourself moments of Body Pride and Sensual Pleasure. Check off each one that appeals to you.

You have created four Power Grind Ins and have trained your brain to honor, celebrate, and enjoy your body and yourself. You are learning how to free yourself from circuits encoded in the past, and welcome a new chapter in your life that will be your best yet!

Body Pride Moments

☐ **Celebrate your Hair:** Style it, cut it, change it!

☐ **Honor your Eyebrows:** Brush them, move them, admire them.

☐ **Check out your Face:** Pull your ears, wiggle your nose, smile wide.

☐ **Ah, that Neck. Oh, those Shoulders:** Strong, gorgeous, sexy!

☐ **Perfect arms. Just right for you:** Perfect for giving hugs.

☐ **Super sturdy Pecs:** Strong and lean, soft and welcoming.

☐ **Good Hands:** Great fingers, nice knuckles, capable in every way.

☐ **Nice Torso there:** Nicely rounded, like a washboard, gorgeous!

☐ **Flex your Biceps:** Strut your stuff, show it off, be strong.

☐ **A great Behind:** Round and wonderful, jiggling and exciting!

☐ **Oh, those Thighs:** Soft to the touch, alluring, muscles galore!

☐ **Good looking Knees:** Square, rounded, fleshy, fantastic!

☐ **Fond of your Feet:** Toes that wiggle, new shoes, nice ankles.

☐ **Decorate Yourself:** Try out new looks, update your style.

☐ **Stand with Body Pride:** Shoulders back, stand tall, feel pride!

☐ **The whole package:** Look in a mirror. You are a great specimen!

☐ **Feel gratitude:** Feel grateful for your body.

☐ **Curl up to sleep:** Feel pride in your body and yourself.

Sensual Pleasure Moments

☐ **Awaken to Sensual Pleasure:** how does your skin feel on the sheets? Stroke your body with love.

☐ **Morning Stretch:** notice how great you feel when you stretch your arms and legs.

☐ **Enjoy your food:** the smell and taste of it, and how it feels to swallow it.

☐ **Water Play:** Be aware of the shower or bath water on your skin. What pleasure!

☐ **Dress with body pride:** Choose clothes that bring you joy and have fun with your appearance.

☐ **Sensual dressing:** As you clothe yourself, be aware of your sensory pleasure.

☐ **Walk intentionally:** Move your body with pride, enjoying each step.

☐ **Use your fingertips wisely:** Pass your fingertips over your hand, thigh, calf, cheek. Wonderful!

☐ **Massage your neck:** Place your hand on the back of your neck (think oxytocin release!) and rub!

☐ **Be aware of your genitals:** We are sexual beings and celebrating our passion, desire, and capacity for pleasure is exciting.

☐ **Sit with body pride:** Sit up tall in your chair and enjoy being present.

☐ **Get to One:** Take a sensuality break, a minute to appreciate your body.

☐ **Move with joy:** Be grateful for your arms, legs, belly, hips – all of you!

☐ **Find one muscle on your body:** Even a finger. Delight in your strength!

☐ **Put your hands over your eyes and smile:** It feels GOOD!

Success Check Day 24

- **Daily Success**

☐ I continued my Joy Practice with 10 Check Ins and 10 Joy Points.

☐ I reset my lifestyle in these nine ways: Exercise, Joy Breakfast, Sanctuary Time, Joy Lunch, Balancing Sleep, Natural Pleasure Binge, Joy Dinner, Body Pride, and Sensual Pleasure.

☐ I made one or more community connections for support with my lifestyle reset.

- **Did I pass the Success Check?   YES   NO**

If you did not, stay with this activity for one more day, then move on.

- **My Amazing Learning:**

_____

- **My Biggest Accomplishment:**

_____

- **My Biggest Challenge:**

_____

Congratulations!

**You have completed Day 24 of The Joy Challenge.
Your next step is Day 25. Jumpstart Raising Your Set Point.**

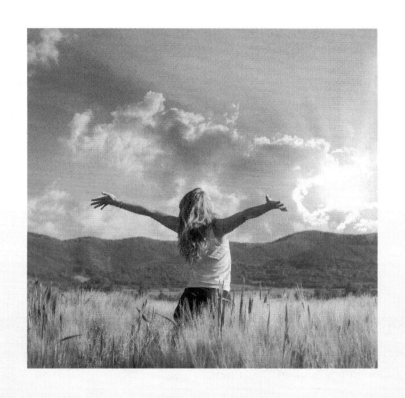

Celebrate Your Joy

Day 25. Jumpstart
Raising Your Set Point

Today we will launch the completion of the Joy Challenge, and move along toward making these changes solid and raising the brain's emotional set point.

We will strengthen our core connection to ourselves in three steps. We'll update how we view Brain State 5, add a meditation to our EBT Practice that encodes the core circuits of emotional evolution, and turn our attention to becoming wired at One.

**It's time to strengthen your core
and raise your set point.**

Why

We are going to create a secure base inside and raise our set point. Our innate biology instills in us a hunger to be at One, and to use our energies to make the world a better place.

The joy of the human condition is that we have a brain that enables us to think magnificent thoughts – to do things for the right reasons – and to self-administer a surge of neurotransmitters for doing it. Learning how to train our brain to accomplish that is not only essential to the survival of the species, but it brings us profound pleasure, the elevated emotions of love, compassion, gratitude, hope, forgiveness, awe, and joy.

In his book, *Spiritual Evolution*, George Vaillant, a Harvard professor, research psychiatrist, and pioneer in human development, describes a special area in the emotional brain: the septal area. It is famous for giving us the ability to have an endless and even addictive drive to please ourselves. However, this area is also activated to bring pleasure from a thought of higher purpose. Our brain gives us the power to activate surges of neurochemicals that reward us in ways that artificial pleasures never could. We can have paradise inside by using our brain well.

My set point is already moving up. My brain randomly triggers a Brain State 5 and I shrug it off. I see a glimmer of joy, then I feel awash in joy. That is not the person I was 30 days ago. I want to keep going.

I can feel my neocortex taking charge. It is highly effective at checking out the wires that are triggered, liking them, and either using them or switching them off. It likes the tools and being aware of my purpose right in the moment – even right now. What's my purpose in saying this? Authenticity.

How

Take three steps to strengthen your core and move from focusing on problems to focusing on higher-order purpose. These are specific actions that help the circuitry in our brain change, so this natural transition becomes smoother and faster.

Step 1. Update the 5 Tool

In the past, when we would go to Brain State 5, our residue from random moments of stress (brain glitches), would take control. We'd activate a Mood Circuit, trigger a Food or Body Circuit, or distance or merge in relationships.

Now we have four Power Grind Ins so these circuits are largely under our control. However, the 5 State remains our pathway to ongoing improvement of our set point. We must reset our relationship with Brain State 5 in order to evolve.

Update your approach to Brain State 5
• This is a Productive 5 State!
• Brain State 5 is part of the process.
• If I can love myself at 5, I can do anything!
• Brain State 5 is a Moment of Opportunity.
• At 5, I connect with the spiritual.
• Before Brain State 1 comes a moment at 5.

So, we must update our 5 Tool. We must say a few words that clearly announce that this state is good for us! Experiment with different phrases until one feels good to you. Then slip in your personal phrase prior to using the 5 Tool. If you bring up a strong nurturing voice and connect with yourself in those moments, Brain State 5 is productive. It will deepen your self-compassion. Oxytocin is higher in that state, perhaps a sign of grace, making it easier to connect with ourselves and the spiritual in challenging moments.

As the brain is highly plastic then, even a tiny bit of self-compassion is strongly remembered. That experience helps us move up our set point. In a way, stress is the new joy!

**Brain State 5 moments are fantastic.
I use them to strengthen my core.**

Step 2. Use the Core Grind In
Core Grind In is a fundamental practice of EBT. Take about five minutes each day to read the seven circuits of emotional evolution. It includes the fundamental expectations of life, the essential pain we must face to accept it, and the rewards we receive from doing so. This practice strengthens our secure connection to ourselves and access to the seven rewards. Each word in the Core Grind In has specific meanings, so please read about them, and personalize the Core Grind In, as needed:

Sanctuary – Peace and Power from Within
I do exist asserts that we are alive. If we recognize that we are alive, we must face our separateness. No matter how much we love others and how much they love us, **we are alone** in that the responsibility for how we use our gift of life resides with us and us alone. By facing our aloneness, we are motivated to cultivate a rich inner life, a **Sanctuary** within us, so we have peace and power from within.

Authenticity – Feeling Whole and Being Genuine
I am not bad means that we have overcome the drive for stress to "split" us and make us think that we are either all good or all bad. When we face the essential pain that **we are not perfect**, we relax, access humility, and feel whole. We can be genuine and experience **Authenticity** in our daily life.

Vibrancy – Healthy with a Zest for Life
I do have power means that we are neither powerless nor all-powerful, either of which leads to suffering and health problems. We face the essential pain that **we are not in complete control** and access far more energy to be healthy with a zest for life, that is, **Vibrancy**.

Integrity – Doing the Right Thing

I can do good means that we are industrious and can take purposeful initiative. When we face the essential pain that **it takes work**, we stop blaming ourselves for the many "failures" and the inevitable pain involved in growth. We stop blaming others too, for life takes work for all of us. No one gets a free ride. The reward is **Integrity**, that gut feeling that we are doing the right thing.

The first four circuits of emotional evolution form the basis for intimacy with self and a secure connection within. Only with that security within can we safely and effectively expand and connect in more profound ways through Intimacy, Spirituality, and Freedom.

Intimacy – Giving and Receiving Love

I can love means that we have accepted that our nature is to love, and we have enough to give to others. The essential pain as we give love is that **some people may reject us**. Although that may hurt, we can take the risk of loving others because we have a secure base within (the first four circuits). Our reward is **Intimacy** in the form that it takes at the time.

Spirituality – Aware of the Grace, Beauty, and Mystery of Life

I am worthy means that we are functional enough to give back to the world. We have evolved enough to give back for the greater good and face the essential pain that **we must receive**. Asking for support from the spiritual as we define it or the greater good stops the overcontrol of outcome that blocks joy. That essential step of humility opens us to experience more of the grace, beauty, and mystery of life, that is, **Spirituality**.

The Core Grind In
7 Circuits to Strengthen Your Core
State this daily to strengthen your core.

Reasonable Expectation	Essential Pain	Earned Reward
I do exist.	I am alone.	Sanctuary
I am not bad.	I am not perfect.	Authenticity
I do have power.	I am not in complete control.	Vibrancy
I can do good.	It takes work.	Integrity
I can love.	Some people may reject me.	Intimacy
I am worthy.	I must receive.	Spirituality
I can have joy.	I must give.	Freedom

Freedom – Common Excesses Fade and We Move Forward in Life

I can have joy means that instead of despairing, we are in hopeful anticipation of the next amazing thing that will happen in our lives. We open ourselves to using our talents in just the way that completes our lives. That takes facing the essential pain that **we must give** at a deeper level. Only then will the whole range of common excesses fade and bring to us the reward of **Freedom**.

Please experiment with this Core Grind In at least once each day. Whether it becomes part of your daily practice or you use it as a "run through" now and then on your way home in the evening, it can be connecting and grounding. What's more, it primes the brain for Advanced EBT and raising your emotional set point.

Share the Core Grind In during connections
I have a weekly connection on Fridays at 8 a.m., and one of us reads the Core Grind In to the other. We have it memorized now. I feel closer to my buddy because we do this.

Use the Core Grind In when you are at Brain State 5
My Mood Circuit is numbing. Sometimes I don't want to deal with my feelings. This Grind In helps a lot. I say it to myself, and it has a stabilizing effect. It can even make my food cravings go away. It helps me put whatever I was worrying about in perspective.

Use it in meditation, prayer, or Sanctuary Time
My morning routine is to check in with myself. Usually, I say a prayer, feel my feelings, and commit to creating joy in my life that day. I use the Core Grind In as a way of focusing on what matters to me: these seven rewards.

Create your own ways to use it, such as a Family Grind In
I sing this Grind In to my three children when we are driving, and they are arguing. They always calm down. Now my 10-year-old is telling me that he is kind to his friends out of integrity. We keep it light and fun, and it is working.

Step 3. Reset your focus: raising your set point
The most powerful thing anyone can do is raise their set point. Whatever situations arise in your day, consider them opportunities to raise your set point and become wired for joy. Think in terms of your Check Ins, Spiral Ups, Power Grind Ins, and Joy Points. Be aware of the earned reward upon which you base each of your actions throughout the day.

I am interested in the reward of Sanctuary right now. My mind is turning to peace and power from within. I want to grab hold of my Power Grind Ins and use them for freedom from overeating. I want all seven rewards, so I have an ever-deepening experience of life. I want to be wired at One, and then after that, deepen my One.

By taking these three steps – updating your 5 Tool, using the Core Grind In, and resetting your focus to raising your set point, you are tapping into the perfection of your emotional brain. What could be more powerful than that?

Success Check Day 25

- **Daily Success**

☐ I continued my Joy Practice with 10 Check Ins and 10 Joy Points.

☐ I updated my 5 Tool, used the Core Grind In, and reset my focus to raising my set point.

☐ I made one or more community connections for support with these activities.

- **Did I pass the Success Check?   YES   NO**

If you did not, stay with this activity for one more day, then move on.

- **My Amazing Learning:**

_____

- **My Biggest Accomplishment:**

_____

- **My Biggest Challenge:**

_____

Wonderful Work!

You have completed Day 25 of The Joy Challenge.
Your next step is Day 26. Tell Your New Story.

Day 26. Tell Your New Story

Throughout the Joy Challenge, you have been gaining insight into your story. The next step of this joy celebration is to create a new story from what you have learned. The story of your weight and eating is a beautiful one, as it makes perfect sense that you would have had just this motivation to clear away stress and return to your joy.

Why

Your journey will continue as you raise your emotional set point and your brain becomes wired for joy, but it is important to pause and reflect about where you have been, where you are now, and where you are going. By telling your emotional brain a new story and encoding that story in your thinking brain, you will not only celebrate your achievements in this book but prepare a clearer pathway to being wired at One.

You might wonder why having a struggle with eating and weight could be perfect. Our set point is the most important predictor of our health and longevity. The set point rises as we evolve emotionally. The lower our set point, the more the brain tries to find easy ways to feel safe and rewarded. We are like children, without a capacity to defer gratification or activate a surge of neurotransmitters because of thoughts of higher purpose. We are still "good" people, but our brain function makes our responses more primitive. What helps us raise our set point? Responding to life's challenges, and using our tools to stay connected to the deepest part of ourselves. That trains our brain for resilience and helps us accept the essential pain of life. It trains our brain to step into negative emotions, and come out the other side of that experience with positive emotions.

Often circuits that trigger overeating and promote weight gain or holding onto extra weight are encoded during times of stress overload or trauma. The circuits act like a "knot" in the brain. Every time we come close to activating that knot of circuits, we go to Brain State 5, and do not rewire them, and often, we make them stronger. We do not do that consciously. The brain perceives that knot of circuits as learnings that keep us alive. We did not die when that knot was encoded, so the information stored in it must be valuable! What's so special about eating and weight is that they are both extremely sensitive to stress. We cannot overcome these problems until we clear away these knots from the past. Often they are bigger than knots. They feel like boulders! They include one or more glitches and can even include quite a few "feel bad" wires. This is one reason that raising our set point is so important, as we clear away these wires layer by layer over time, until we "move" that boulder! When we do, two things happen. One, we stop overeating and release extra weight with joy if these changes have eluded us. Two, each Cycle we do to clear that boulder or untie that knot is a blessing! Hidden in that circuit is a kernel of wisdom, and because we have felt our feelings as we have revealed it, we have far more empathy for others and compassion for ourselves. In other words, rewiring the brain to have freedom from food and weight issues enables us to grow, evolve, mature, and know ourselves at a deeper level. It is not unusual for people to experience a spiritual deepening and become far more aware of the sacred meaning of their life. Adversity leads to maturity. Side-stepping feelings and eating does not bring us the same rewards. The process can be slow at times, but I know of no other way to access an abundance of the seven rewards of a purposeful life, and your experience of moving past eating and weight issues is bound to be one of the most rewarding and glorious experiences of your life. I know it has been for mine.

How

Complete the My New Story activity that follows, then tell your story to yourself and share it by reading it aloud to yourself, sharing it with your group if you are participating in one, or savoring it in a moment of connection with someone who is special to you!

My family was very loving but had a lot of challenges. My sister was a year younger than I was and she was so adorable that I felt invisible and left out. I don't know when I encoded my Food Circuit, but I wouldn't be surprised if it was about the time my sister was born. I remember my parents complaining that I dropped her a lot! My Mood Circuit came on when I was nine and dealing with early breast development and having no idea what was going on in my body. Nobody talked with me about it and I had a Distancing Circuit by then so I let it go. I ate more, and my mother, who was a vegan and skinny, was horrified that I was SO BIG, which delighted me. My weight was perfect because I didn't have to deal with my sister or parents and could eat my way into being so heavy that I completely frustrated them. It took two decades before I realized that nobody cared how fat I was or how much I ate. I was not happy with my resulting food addiction and then I found EBT. I am taking responsibility for my wires and learning how to rewire the past and climb up to new heights. My reason for raising my set point is freedom. It's more than freedom from stress eating or weight, it's freedom from carrying forward their wires. I love my family, but I want a life of joy and rewards, and if I decide to have children, I want to pass along joy wires to them.

Your story will take its own form, but notice as you write it that you have complete compassion for yourself. The past makes sense, the present is perfect, and the future seems . . . exciting! Retell the story of your food and weight that makes it clear why your entire history has made perfect sense! This is a healing experience and important for the next step of beginning to raise your set point for lasting improvements in the quality of your life.

My New Story

In the Past . . .

In the past, OF COURSE I would have the drives to overeat and hold onto extra weight, because of these circuits:

A Food Circuit that told me that . . .

I got my _____ from _____.

A Mood Circuit that told me that . . .

I got my _____ from _____.

A Love Circuit that told me that . . .

I got my _____ from _____.

A Body Circuit that told me that . . .

I got my _____ from _____.

It is highly effective to write the detail of circuit discovery process. Please journal the story of the circuits that blocked your joy.

In the Present . . .

Now I have discovered and have begun to transform my:

- ☐ Food Circuit

- ☐ Mood Circuit

- ☐ Love Circuit

- ☐ Body Circuit

Please write the story of the ways that you are creating more joy in your life now.

In the Future . . .

I will use my Power Grind Ins to transform these circuits and continue my EBT Practice until I have an abundance of:

- ☐ Sanctuary
- ☐ Authenticity
- ☐ Vibrancy
- ☐ Integrity
- ☐ Intimacy
- ☐ Spirituality
- ☐ Freedom

Please write the story of the ways that you will create more joy in the future as you transform these circuits.

The Perfection of My Brain

Now that you have told the new story of your eating and weight, please reflect on the ways that rewiring your brain to have freedom from food and weight issues has helped you evolve. Each rewiring delivers a kernel of wisdom and raises your set point. Empathy is only derived from a deep connection to ourselves, and each rewiring deepens our inner security and emotional depth. Please describe how overcoming food and weight issues has enhanced the quality of your life.

Success Check Day 26

- **Daily Success**

☐ I continued my Joy Practice with 10 Check Ins and 10 Joy Points.

☐ I told the new story of my food and weight.

☐ I made one or more community connections for support with my story.

- **Did I pass the Success Check?   YES   NO**

If you did not, stay with this activity for one more day, then move on.

- **My Amazing Learning:**

_____

- **My Biggest Accomplishment:**

_____

- **My Biggest Challenge:**

_____

Congratulations!

**You have completed Day 26 of The Joy Challenge.
Your next step is Day 27. The Vibrancy Plan Day 1.**

Day 27. The Vibrancy Plan Day 1

Today we will begin the three-day culminating experience for the Joy Challenge.

You will apply everything you have learned in this book to check in with yourself, then stay connected to yourself and adopt a healthy, vibrant lifestyle. In addition, you will take five-minute Power Breaks four times daily to use your Power Grind Ins. They will make it far easier for you to transform those circuits into new ones that will give you the drives to eat healthy and experience natural, lasting weight loss.

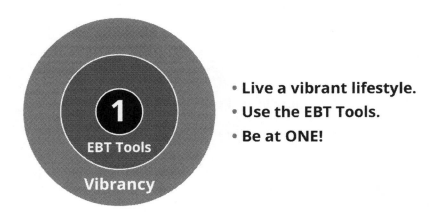

* **Live a vibrant lifestyle.**
* **Use the EBT Tools.**
* **Be at ONE!**

Why

We need a "Vibrancy Reset" in which we not only check in but stay checked in. By weaving a commitment to a healthy lifestyle into your plan, sustaining that new way of life becomes far easier. We feel charged up and motivated!

I did not know how great I could feel. Now that I have experienced it, I want more of this. My reptile wants me to return to my old stagnant, stressed life. Nope. There is no way I'm going to do that!

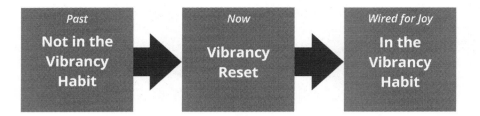

Past		Now		Wired for Joy
Not in the Vibrancy Habit	→	**Vibrancy Reset**	→	**In the Vibrancy Habit**

How

It's easy! Today as well as for the next two days, the day's learning includes a checklist of activities for a day of vibrancy. First, modify the plan to meet your needs, and then use the checklist as you move through your day. You don't have to do this perfectly to see important results.

Think of this as a time to feast on natural pleasures and outsmart the reptilian brain's drives to keep you addicted to stress. Instead, connect with your inherent strength, goodness, and wisdom. Be at One!

I chose exercise I love, which is walking my dog. And I did Sanctuary Time when I got home from work. I went into my bedroom, shut off the light, and curled up in a ball on my bed. I did Cycles in my head and got to One. Dinner was not the usual pasta, bread, and ice cream, but instead a plate of greens, avocados, chicken, and plenty of olive oil. It was delicious. My natural pleasure binge topped it off!

The Vibrancy Plan Day 1

- Read The Vibrancy Plan checklist for Day 1.
- Personalize the plan to meet your needs.
- Enjoy your first day of vibrancy!

Make it Easy

Eat for vibrancy

Establish a pattern of eating that is in harmony with the lifestyle of our hunter-gatherer ancestors, the one that our genes evolved to prefer. The EBT 3-Point Food Plan involves three evidence-based practices: eating only when hungry, eating mainly Joy Foods, and taking a 12-hour food rest. Emphasize lean protein, healthy fats, and fiber foods because most people who eat them are satisfied for longer and have fewer blood sugar lows. Add enough Stress Foods to avoid feeling deprived.

Build on your five lifestyle resets

All five of the lifestyle resets as well as your Joy Practice balance your dopamine. It is essential to ending overeating and releasing extra weight to become hooked on natural pleasure. Sugar is mildly addictive (at least), and the brain needs more and more of it to feel good. Meanwhile, both sugary diets and obesity can "burn out" some dopamine receptors so that it is harder to feel good without a big wallop of an artificial reward. The point is to have freedom, and by making these small but important changes in lifestyle to promote natural pleasure, the zest for life returns!

Be sure to personalize your plan. Speed it up and do everything on the list or take a more gradual approach and implement fewer of them. However, err on the side of doing more, as you will feel so much better that you will want to continue it.

When I thought of putting this all together, I was excited and scared. Then I used the plan – imperfectly but well – and now I feel better than I have in years.

Why dopamine matters!

Dopamine is our "get up and go" reward chemical.
Natural pleasures promote healthy dopamine levels,
whereas artificial pleasures trigger extremes.

"I feast on natural pleasure to balance my dopamine."

Take Power Breaks!

It's essential to keep the Stress Triangle in check so that your reward and stress centers make it easy to enjoy natural pleasures, eat healthy, and begin to release weight with joy. You now have your four Power Grind Ins, so take five minutes at regular intervals throughout the day to zap those circuits and activate your reward center. You can change your chemistry naturally! Give yourself a dose of healthy chemicals during your Power Breaks and experience how easy it is to live a vibrant lifestyle.

Imagine yourself choosing to activate these healing chemicals throughout the day by using the tools. Also, notice the impact of taking a five-minute Power Break four times today, as you'll identify your amazing learning about using them tomorrow.

Use the checklist on the next page to guide your way. As always, make it fun!

Success Check Day 27
The Vibrancy Plan Checklist: Day 1

Today, I . . .

☐ Created my day when I awoke: "I am creating joy in my life"

☐ Made a community connection

☐ Exercised for 10 to 30 minutes in the morning

☐ Ate a Joy Breakfast and drank one or two glasses of water

☐ Did meaningful work in the morning

☐ Ate a Joy Lunch and drank one or two glasses of water

☐ Did meaningful work in the afternoon

☐ Exercised for 10 to 30 minutes in the afternoon or evening

☐ Took Sanctuary Time for 10 minutes

☐ Ate a Joy Dinner and drank one or two glasses of water

☐ Had a natural pleasure binge

☐ Made another community connection

☐ Took a food rest for 12 hours

☐ Created my day at bedtime: "I am creating joy in my life"

☐ Enjoyed balancing sleep for eight hours

Be aware of your EBT practice of Check Ins, Joy Points, and Power Breaks:

Did I check in 10 times?   YES   NO

Did I score 10 Joy Points?   YES   NO

Did I take four Power Breaks?   YES   NO

Total the number of activities you checked in the list above:

Total Vibrancy Points Today _____

<8 = low vibrancy   8-12 = moderate vibrancy   >12 = high vibrancy

My Vibrancy Day 1:   LOW   MODERATE   HIGH

- **My Amazing Learning:**

_____

- **My Biggest Accomplishment:**

_____

- **My Biggest Challenge:**

_____

Congratulations!

You have completed Day 27 of The Joy Challenge.
Your next step is Day 28. The Vibrancy Plan Day 2.

Day 28. The Vibrancy Plan Day 2

Great work completing the Vibrancy Plan Day 1. You are now in the second day of your Vibrancy Reset.

You are using both your brain state and your lifestyle to improve the chemical cascade that reduces your stress and activates surges of feel-good chemicals like dopamine, serotonin, endorphins, and oxytocin and to separate yourself from the stress-infested, addicted world we live in. Instead of living with these addictive drives (all 5 Circuits are addictions), we are using lifestyle and rewiring to gain more freedom in our lives. This is your opportunity to begin to break free of the stress cycle!

Check to see if you need to increase your Vibrancy Points (be even healthier) or decrease them (ease up a bit). Use your brain state as a guide. Some stress shows that you are changing; too much stress is counterproductive.

Why

Checking in and adjusting your plan is really important, in part because the missing piece of information is how your Power Breaks work.

The Vibrancy Plan Day 2

- Read The Vibrancy Plan checklist for Day 2.
- Personalize the plan to meet your needs.
- Enjoy your second day of vibrancy!

If your Power Breaks are short-circuiting stress and stopping cravings and unwanted drives, then your stress level will be significantly lower. You have more power to change, without triggering a protracted Brain State 5. If you have more bandwidth, then use it!

I forgot to do the Power Breaks during Day 1, and it still worked pretty well. I was running at Brain States 1 to 3 yesterday. It was a great day. I'm going to take four Power Breaks today, and see how much they help.

Err on the side of taking more Power Breaks, in addition to living a vibrant lifestyle, to break all four circuits as quickly as possible. When you break all four circuits, the joy of releasing unneeded weight can kick in. Weight loss is what improves your brain's leptin sensitivity the most. Increased leptin sensitivity is a powerful appetite suppressant and freedom-from-hunger booster.

Why leptin matters!

Leptin is a "stop-eating" chemical that shuts off appetite.
Obesity and high insulin levels derail leptin,
causing chronic hunger and weight gain.

"I eat Joy Foods to keep my leptin on track."

Take your Power Break Inventory for Day 1

Check whether or not you used each of your four Power Grind Ins during your five-minute Power Breaks throughout the day yesterday.

Notice if you used all of them or were drawn to focusing on one. Everyone is different. Some people use all four each time; others home in on one or two. Experiment. Which way helps you change faster? Your Power Grind Ins will help you win the war against the reptile. It will calm down as you move through Advanced EBT, but it is always a force to be contended with.

I used my Mood and Food Power Grind Ins during the day because they help me keep my food cravings away. But I noticed in the evening I needed all four of my Grind Ins. I am having fun singing them and using funny voices and they are working!

How

Today, check if you want to speed it up, slow it down, or keep the plan the same. You may find the second day more challenging, experiencing some detox from the artificial rewards of your previous lifestyle. Flexibility is key. Do not do more than you can. Triggering a protracted 5 State is not the plan – it's not fun or effective.

Plan your Power Breaks at regular intervals throughout the day. You can say your Power Grind Ins to yourself or aloud. Either way, the more passion in your voice, the more emotional amplification you have, the more your wires will change!

I go into the restroom, find a stall, and sit there for five minutes. Nobody sees my face, which is very animated, or that I am waving my arms around. I am completely committed to breaking all four wires in the second 30 days, and I want to get a head start NOW.

I use my Power Breaks as a form of Sanctuary Time. I have two stepchildren and a baby and no time to myself. I feel great about taking the four breaks because it impacts my wires, which means it impacts their wires. I'm going to transform my wires for myself and for my family.

The most important outcome from today's plan is for you to know more about how you want to live. Which elements of the plan make life better for you, and which are not realistic or helpful?

Use the checklist on the next page to personalize your plan. It must be fun or you will not stick with it. Enjoy this second day of vibrancy!

Success Check Day 28
The Vibrancy Plan Checklist: Day 2

Today, I . . .

- ☐ Created my day when I awoke: "I am creating joy in my life"
- ☐ Made a community connection
- ☐ Exercised for 10 to 30 minutes in the morning
- ☐ Ate a Joy Breakfast and drank one or two glasses of water
- ☐ Did meaningful work in the morning
- ☐ Ate a Joy Lunch and drank one or two glasses of water
- ☐ Did meaningful work in the afternoon
- ☐ Exercised for 10 to 30 minutes in the afternoon or evening
- ☐ Took Sanctuary Time for 10 minutes
- ☐ Ate a Joy Dinner and drank one or two glasses of water
- ☐ Had a natural pleasure binge
- ☐ Made another community connection
- ☐ Took a food rest for 12 hours
- ☐ Created my day at bedtime: "I am creating joy in my life"
- ☐ Enjoyed balancing sleep for eight hours

Be aware of your EBT practice of Check Ins, Joy Points, and Power Breaks:

Did I check in 10 times?   YES   NO

Did I score 10 Joy Points?   YES   NO

Did I take four Power Breaks?   YES   NO

Total the number of activities you checked in the list above

Total Vibrancy Points Today_____

<8=low vibrancy   8-12=moderate vibrancy   >12=high vibrancy

My Vibrancy Day 2: LOW   MODERATE HIGH

- **My Amazing Learning:**

_____

- **My Biggest Accomplishment:**

_____

- **My Biggest Challenge:**

_____

Congratulations!

You have completed Day 28 of The Joy Challenge.
Your next step is Day 29. The Vibrancy Plan Day 3.

Day 29. The Vibrancy Plan Day 3

As you complete three days of vibrancy, you can transition into using a personalized version of this plan for the next 30 days. This is a moment of opportunity, as incorporating a vibrant lifestyle and transforming these hefty Stress Circuits can lead to a brain and body reset.

The Power Breaks and the natural pleasure binges are winning me over. This is a great way to live!

Today is your last day of the 3-Day Vibrancy Plan, your reset to a more vibrant lifestyle of natural pleasures that delivers a zest for life. Check how your Power Grind Ins are working, and ask for support for the second 30 days of the program.

Why
The reptile lies in wait. You will be using your prefrontal cortex to deactivate the Stress Circuits stored in the amygdala consistently for 30 days. In a very brief period, you can make solid the amazing work you have done in this challenge!

We're going to do this the fun way. We'll focus on feasting on natural pleasures, living a vibrant life, and collecting so many Joy Points that it is all . . . easy!

The Vibrancy Plan Day 3
- Read The Vibrancy Plan checklist for Day 3.
- Check how your Power Grind Ins are working.
- Identify your support needs.

I want freedom from all these stress circuit addictions. I came to EBT for food, but I am now committed to creating joy in my life. I have seen what stress and addictions do to people – even soft addictions like merging. That's not the life I want for myself. Count me in!

Why endorphins matter!

A natural morphine that surges after dopamine
motivates us to take action, endorphins bring
euphoria and a sense of optimal well-being.

"My euphoria is non-addictive. I use Joy Points."

Take your Power Circuit Inventory for Day 2

Notice which of the four Power Grind Ins you used yesterday, and which ones worked. Your brain and your Power Grind Ins are unique, so the best indicator of the ideal way to use these Power Grind Ins is how using them impacts you.

If one is not helping, update the Power Grind In or try using it at a different time. Experiment. What is the goal? Breaking those circuits. You will know when you have broken them. The attachment to unhealthy eating is gone, the love affair is over, the excesses become like old news. They may even fade from your memory.

I think this is working! I posted all my Power Grind Ins on the fridge. I have been using them in the evenings, all four of them in a row, and I have not been overeating at night! I am not forcing myself not to. I just don't want to! And I think I even like the food rest! Amazing!

How

For Day 3, check if you want to speed it up, slow it down, or keep the plan the same. Reflect on what you are learning from these three days, and how the Power Break schedule is working for you. Make any needed changes and consider how important it is for you to access support to make this plan work.

No lone islands – ask for support

As you begin the second 30 days of the program, your brain will integrate the vast changes you have made during the first 30 days. During this period of intensive reconsolidating, you will be consistent (but not rigidly so) and passionate. You will be determined, focused, and excited about feasting on natural pleasures and watching your drive to eat when you are not hungry fade away.

You have worked so hard to complete the 30-Day Joy Challenge that this is your time to cash in on your earnings. If you fold now, you will miss out on a life-changing experience.

It is essential that you arrange for support. Relationships are two-way streets, so just the way you help others, they can help you. As your set point rises because of your vibrancy, others around you "catch" your higher state. Helping you, in time, helps them.

I told my boyfriend that I am going to get up earlier and go to the gym, so I can't do errands in the morning. He said okay. I was afraid to ask him (my Merge Circuit operating), but I did it anyway. He didn't like it, but he will like my zest for life down the road.

Sometimes asking for support is not met with joy. Most people like things to stay the same and if you are taking more time for your vibrancy, it may mean more work for them. Most of us over-give to those around us and these folks (quite naturally) like it.

My teenage son groaned when I told him he'd have to cook dinner for the rest of us on Tuesdays and Thursdays, so that I would have more time to take care of myself. He made it sound like I was the worst father on Earth. Then he started cooking and he was great at it. He is proud of himself, and I am at One when I come home those nights.

Use the checklist on the next page and reflect on your Vibrancy Plan Day 3 and fine-tune your plan. Keep it flexible, but clear, so that you know what you intend to do going forward. Make it challenging enough so that after 30 days, your Vibrancy Habit will help you move up your set point more quickly and easily.

This is your time

Everyone has a time when change is in the wind and they can succeed. You have made it this far in the Joy Challenge. Just by sticking with this exceedingly challenging course, I know for sure that this is your time.

Build on your momentum now and challenge your perceptions. You can have more joy, more power, and more freedom than you ever imagined possible! Stay the course!

Success Check Day 29
The Vibrancy Plan Checklist: Day 3

Today, I . . .

☐ Created my day when I awoke: "I am creating joy in my life"

☐ Made a community connection

☐ Exercised for 10 to 30 minutes in the morning

☐ Ate a Joy Breakfast and drank one or two glasses of water

☐ Did meaningful work in the morning

☐ Ate a Joy Lunch and drank one or two glasses of water

☐ Did meaningful work in the afternoon

☐ Exercised for 10 to 30 minutes in the afternoon or evening

☐ Took Sanctuary Time for 10 minutes

☐ Ate a Joy Dinner and drank one or two glasses of water

☐ Had a natural pleasure binge

☐ Made another community connection

☐ Took a food rest for 12 hours

☐ Created my day at bedtime: "I am creating joy in my life"

☐ Enjoyed balancing sleep for eight hours

Be aware of your EBT practice of Check Ins, Joy Points, and Power Breaks:

Did I check in 10 times?   YES   NO

Did I score 10 Joy Points?   YES   NO

Did I take four Power Breaks?   YES   NO

Total the number of activities you checked in the list above:

Total Vibrancy Points Today _____

<8=low vibrancy   8-12=moderate vibrancy   >12=high vibrancy

My Vibrancy Day 3:   LOW   MODERATE   HIGH

- **My Amazing Learning:**

_____

- **My Biggest Accomplishment:**

_____

- **My Biggest Challenge:**

_____

Congratulations!

You have completed Day 29 of The Joy Challenge.
Your next step is Day 30. Celebrate Your Joy.

Day 30. Celebrate Your Joy

In the last 30 days, you have learned how to rewire your own emotional brain. It's time to celebrate what you have accomplished and determine how to make the most of your gains. Please take three steps:

Step 1. Celebrate Your Joy
You have new powers to control your elusive emotional brain. You have learned new tools, and it's time to celebrate that you have completed this foundational course in taking charge of your unconscious mind.

I was tempted to have a hot fudge sundae, but my Food Circuit has already transformed, so hot fudge does not "do it" for me anymore. I went to the nearby hilltop at sunset and was in awe of what I had accomplished.

I celebrated by updating my calendar and committing to more Sanctuary Time. I made a special place for Sanctuary Time in an alcove in my house that is quiet and comforting.

I bought myself new clothes. It was in celebration of my new body pride and feeling connected to the deepest part of myself. YES!!!

Step 2. Commit to Raising Your Set Point
You have done the basic work. The foundation has been built. Now it's time to construct the "house." That's the seven rewards that raise the brain's set point for lasting and profound improvements in food, mood, love, body, and health. This takes as long as it takes but you can complete one course in as little as one month, so consider this a one-year program, however, take longer if you like. The challenge is to commit to becoming wired for JOY, wired at ONE! Consider which of the seven rewards is your ultimate desire . . . and it will motivate you to become wired for joy.

I am not going to quit now. I want to reset my brain, particularly because my children have already acquired some of my wires, and the best way to help them update their wires is for ME to update my own! My ultimate reward is Integrity, doing the right thing.

I'm going to raise my set point, and I know that I need structure and support to do it. I have quit other programs. I'm completely "in" on this and my reward is FREEDOM.

Step 3. Share the Tools

EBT is a movement. The #1 epidemic worldwide is the emotional brain in stress. We have the neuroscience to overcome that stress, and make the challenges we face a positive aspect of our lives. The more stress we face and move through, the more our set point rises. Please share EBT in your own time and own way with at least one person. Become part of EBT's mission in a way that works for you. Give back and become part of the solution that the world most needs right now.

I'm inviting family members to try out the tools for a week. A man in my telegroup is part of a family in which 10 members have an EBT practice. His entire family is becoming more connected and healthier. I want that for my family.

I'm going to share this with my daughter who is nine years old and so anxious. I'm going to teach her the Flow Tool. I think I'll call it the Feelings Game!

Celebrate your new power to create joy in your life

Let's take the Joy Inventory one more time. Changes in all three areas – needs, rewards, and connection – are signs of your raising set point and your enhanced emotional evolution. They are measures of your capacity to experience an exceptional life. Compare your joy to what you experienced at the beginning and middle of this book. Celebrate your progress!

The Joy Inventory

Needs

In the last week, how often did you meet each of your basic needs?

Purpose
  1 = Rarely   2 = Sometimes   3 = Often   4 = Very Often

Pleasure
  1 = Rarely   2 = Sometimes   3 = Often   4 = Very Often

Comfort
  1 = Rarely   2 = Sometimes   3 = Often   4 = Very Often

Love
  1 = Rarely   2 = Sometimes   3 = Often   4 = Very Often

Safety
  1 = Rarely   2 = Sometimes   3 = Often   4 = Very Often

Total Needs Score _____

Rewards

In the last week, how often did you experience these rewards?

Sanctuary: Peace and power from within
  1 = Rarely   2 = Sometimes   3 = Often   4 = Very Often

Authenticity: Feeling whole and being genuine
  1 = Rarely   2 = Sometimes   3 = Often   4 = Very Often

Vibrancy: Healthy with a zest for life
  1 = Rarely   2 = Sometimes   3 = Often   4 = Very Often

Integrity: Doing the right thing
  1 = Rarely   2 = Sometimes   3 = Often   4 = Very Often

Intimacy: Giving and receiving love
  1 = Rarely   2 = Sometimes   3 = Often   4 = Very Often

Spirituality: Aware of the grace, beauty, and mystery of life
  1 = Rarely   2 = Sometimes   3 = Often   4 = Very Often

Freedom: Common excesses fade
  1 = Rarely   2 = Sometimes   3 = Often   4 = Very Often

Total Rewards Score _____

Connection

In the last week, how often did you connect in this way?

Being aware that I can create joy in my life
  1 = Rarely   2 = Sometimes   3 = Often   4 = Very Often

Choosing to create a moment of joy
  1 = Rarely   2 = Sometimes   3 = Often   4 = Very Often

Spiraling up from stress to joy
  1 = Rarely   2 = Sometimes   3 = Often   4 = Very Often

Enjoying sensory pleasures
  1 = Rarely   2 = Sometimes   3 = Often   4 = Very Often

Appreciating the joy of eating healthy
  1 = Rarely   2 = Sometimes   3 = Often   4 = Very Often

Feeling the joy of releasing extra weight
  1 = Rarely   2 = Sometimes   3 = Often   4 = Very Often

Feeling love for myself
  1 = Rarely   2 = Sometimes   3 = Often   4 = Very Often

Feeling love for others
  1 = Rarely   2 = Sometimes   3 = Often   4 = Very Often

Feeling love for all living beings
  1 = Rarely   2 = Sometimes   3 = Often   4 = Very Often

Total Connection Score _____

The Joy Inventory Summary

Category	Baseline Score	Current Score	Progress	Joy Range
Needs	_____	_____	_____	15 to 20
Rewards	_____	_____	_____	21 to 28
Connection	_____	_____	_____	27 to 36
Total	_____	_____	_____	63 to 84

What is your amazing learning about your needs?

_____

What is your amazing learning about your rewards?

_____

What is your amazing learning about your connection?

_____

Moving forward

After celebrating your accomplishments in this course, you can build on them with 30 days of a brain reset. Your brain needs to reorganize around the major changes you have made, making the new circuitry dominant and solid.

You can focus on transforming all four of your Stress Circuits and train your basal ganglia for a vibrant lifestyle. Then we'll move on to the first reward in Advanced EBT: Sanctuary. Congratulations on completing this course!

Move on to the next chapter to create a sensible and life-changing plan to do the most powerful thing that anyone can do: raise your set point and become wired for joy.

Great Work!

You have completed The Joy Challenge.
Your Next Step is to Become Wired for Joy.

Next Step: Become Wired for Joy

The wires at the bottom of your brain are changing and yet, to make these changes solid requires focused attention and finishing the job.

The challenge is to take 30 days and transform all four circuits and, by staying the course with a flexible, vibrant lifestyle, train your brain in the Vibrancy Habit. After those 30 days, the challenge is to move up your set point until you have reset your brain for a profound state of connection. You can then be wired at One, able to move through all five brain states and sooner or later spiral up to joy.

When we started training people in EBT, we knew that the science showed we should be changing the most fundamental circuits in the emotional brain and certain things should happen as the set point rose. Over time, we began to look for those signs, as when the set point changes, the brain behaves differently in response to the demands of daily life.

We saw that without guided support, the reptilian brain resists and that causes the prefrontal cortex to lose focus on raising the set point. So, we developed the Advanced EBT courses to guide the process in amassing the higher-order rewards of life.

Key steps during the second 30 days

What do you do during the second 30 days? You use the Vibrancy Plan daily and record what you do. Also, use your Power Grind Ins four times daily and track your progress with breaking all four of your circuits.

This honoring requires NOT targeting any more circuits. Instead, break free of the circuits you have identified. Take five minutes four times daily for a Power Break to use your Grind Ins. Each wire is from a different domain of life. Rewiring all four of these major circuits will strengthen your secure base, so you can be present, aware, and connected. Just the way a table is sturdier with four legs than three, be sure to transform all four of your circuits. This strengthens the all-important connection for optimal functioning between your thinking brain and emotional brain (neural integration) so that you can become wired for joy more easily and more rapidly.

Second, stop the Stress Triangle from spinning in the direction of a declining set point, and turn it around so that you are chemically primed to raise your set point by continuing with your Vibrancy Plan. This will not be easy! However, consistently practicing vibrancy for 30 days changes the basal ganglia (the brain's habit center). You will encode the Vibrancy Habit. Research has shown that even if we do not do it perfectly, the repeated use of a simple plan trains the brain to sustain lasting change.

The Second 30 Days

* Make vibrancy a habit.
* Clear away those Stress Circuits.
* Prepare to become wired for joy.

I took a break for the second 30 days, and followed my version of the Vibrancy Plan. I broke all four of my circuits, too. First, my Mood Circuit transformed, which makes me laugh. I was addicted to depression for how many years? I broke my attachment to depression, and now those mood states are annoying, but they pass. Both my eating sweets wire and my distancing circuit are largely gone. The last one I transformed was my Body Circuit, which was judging my height (too tall) and weight (breasts too big). Now I'm ready for Advanced EBT, starting with the Sanctuary course, peace and power from within.

Lasting change is what matters

You are embarking on a journey that was not possible just 10 years ago. As long as we are cornered by these Stress Circuits, we seem to be changing, but instead, we are swapping one excess for another – such as stopping overeating and taking up overworking or overspending.

Lasting change is so rare and powerful that researchers have studied those who have achieved it. We have learned that for weight loss to matter to health it must be lasting. Even losing a small percentage of our weight (ten percent on average) for one year is enough to improve health measures such as blood pressure and to reverse or slow cellular aging, a predictor of heart disease, cancer, and diabetes. By rewiring the powerful circuits in the emotional brain, it's easier to stop overeating and release weight in the short term, and in the longer term, to meaningfully impact the quality of our lives.

Be your own natural chemist – pull your own strings

The most effective way to move forward with releasing weight naturally and ending overeating is to use the EBT Tools to control your own Stress Triangle. When the brain unleashes a Stress Circuit, the chemical surges make us hungry, anxious, depressed, and lethargic. We are chemically-affected (see the Stress Circuit graphic below.)

Stress Circuits
(Allostatic Circuits)

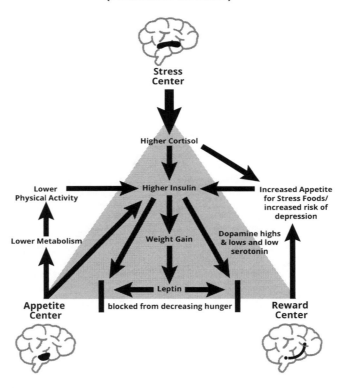

Stress Circuits trigger the Stress Triangle, which activates deleterious chemical surges that promote cravings, anxiety, depression, lethargy, hunger, overeating, and weight gain. Adapted from Mietus-Snyder, M. & Lustig, R., *Annual Review of Medicine* 2008:59:147-162.

On the other hand, if we reach for our tools and short circuit that wire, a Joy Circuit takes control. Soothing chemicals take the lead (see Joy Circuits graphic below). Think of yourself as a chemist, sitting in your thinking brain, fiddling with your chemistry. Want to feel great and release weight? Spiral up to One. Zap a circuit. Pound away at your Power Grind Ins. YOU have amazing power. See the chemical impacts on the graphic below, some immediate and some accruing in time.

Joy Circuits
(Homeostatic Circuits)

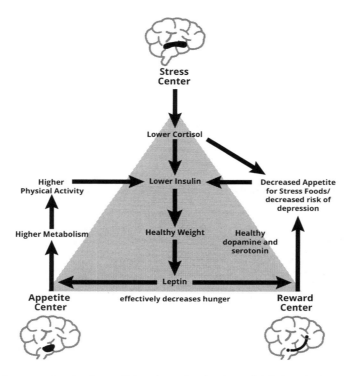

Joy Circuits can calm the Stress Triangle, activating beneficial chemical surges that promote healthy eating, lasting weight loss, and optimal well-being. Adapted from Mietus-Snyder, M. & Lustig, R., *Annual Review of Medicine* 2008:59:147-162. For a review of the science of stress, reward, and appetite, see Robert Lustig's books *Fat Chance* and *The Hacking of the American Mind.*

The fun of this science is that we have new ways to understand ourselves. You might start noticing how different set points, different brain states, and different experiences breaking wires impact your eating and weight. The three aspects of life that are most sensitive to stress are food, weight, and sex. The four top sexual problems in both men and women are stress-sensitive. As stress abates, all three tend to improve. As our emotional brain has no walls, our stress can come from within or be transmitted through social and family relationships.

For example, when my set point drops down when stress is high, I don't like fruit as much. When I move my set point back up, oranges and apples taste delicious. When I became involved with Walt, my merge circuit started acting up ("I get my safety from others") which is common during the "falling in love" stage of a relationship, when dopamine surges cause us to bond. Also, I must have encoded a Body Circuit, along the lines of "I get my safety from being bigger." Of course, this was completely unconscious, but I noticed that I was holding onto a few extra pounds.

The Joy of Healthy Weight

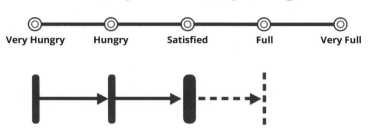

Spiral up to One.
Eat to satisfy your hunger.
Enjoy a natural pleasure binge and
finish with an extra Joy Point!

After a while, with the merging over, when oxytocin surges caused a deepening of connection, I was uncomfortable with that extra weight because it did not authentically reflect who I was. I went after my Body Circuit, and I broke it. With that circuit cleared, my Stress Triangle quieted down, too. Within a week or so, I noticed that I was eating less. Food wasn't so important to me. Feeling slightly hungry felt good to me, a sign that I was releasing weight in support of authenticity, adopting the weight that was right for me. I never lose weight quickly, as I don't think it's good for my whole self. Just think how many wires need to flip from Stress Circuits to Joy Circuits to adjust to a new weight! However, rather rapidly, I felt that "zing" of joy that I was releasing weight and it came off over a period of six weeks or so. It was both fun and easy.

You have been taking charge of that Stress Triangle from the moment you started collecting Joy Points. If you are curious about the science behind EBT, two books authored by endocrinologist and obesity expert Robert Lustig, MD will give you a vast array of scientific information with his characteristic entertaining style. They are *Fat Chance* and *The Hacking of the American Mind*.

Is releasing weight beginning to sound like fun?
You have started to quiet that Stress Triangle that causes overeating. As you take charge of your chemistry through taking charge of your wires, you will feel differently. You are now spontaneously activating and sustaining the activation of homeostatic rather than allostatic circuits. That changes the three major brain centers of the Stress Triangle.

Everyone is different, but this can have an impact on the amygdala (stress center) and the release of the stress hormone cortisol which promotes comfort eating. Cortisol also increases ghrelin, the hunger hormone, which triggers us to start eating, even in the absence of body hunger. With enough change in your circuits, you may eat less often. Cortisol causes extremes of dopamine, which make us crave high-sugar, high-fat foods, the foods that are low in fiber and therefore diminish Peptide YY, the hormone which signals us to stop eating. You may be less hungry and eat less food. Cravings may quiet down too, as dopamine levels normalize. You may begin to have more freedom from thinking about food and seeking to eat in the absence of body hunger.

I carried food with me everywhere and as soon as I had a slight twinge of hunger, I'd eat candy, then 90 minutes later, I'd be in a blood sugar low and starving for more. I stick with Joy Foods now and I'm close to breaking two of my circuits. I can see how addicted I have been to food. I'm sick of that. I want freedom.

As eating Joy Foods and exercising become encoded in your habit center (basal ganglia), other changes can follow. Your cells may become less resistant to insulin, so less insulin is secreted, and it's insulin that clears glucose from the blood and increases hunger. In time, excess insulin (hyperinsulinemia), which causes chronic hunger, as well as anxiety, fatigue, and obesity, can fade.

Over time, that chronic hunger and the tendency to gain weight may diminish. Leptin levels rise with obesity, telling the hypothalamus (appetite center) that you have plenty of fat stores. However, hyperinsulinemia, primarily caused by a Stress Food diet, makes leptin signaling go on the blink. The appetite center doesn't get the message that we aren't starving to death and instead we keep on overeating. However, eating healthy, releasing weight, and exercise can all help increase leptin sensitivity.

What's more, nothing is as impactful as your body pride. Once the switch flips in your brain and you are so overcome with love for yourself, your body, and the gift of life, the Stress Triangle is at your service. It will start spewing those healing chemicals that make releasing weight a joy. You spiral up to One, eat when hungry until the hunger disappears, then feast on natural pleasures (have a pleasure binge) and finish it off with an extra Joy Point. Hunger? Well, a little of it feels encouraging that you are rediscovering a weight that is right for you.

I had been hungry nearly constantly ever since I could remember. I have rewired my unconscious mind and I am in love with my body and myself and the weight is falling off me. It's a miracle.

I had a love affair with food, a food addiction since age 14. It's over. There is no passion left. Food is just food. I am relishing the joy of releasing weight and I love my natural pleasure binges!

I lost the first five pounds after I fried my Food Circuit, then nothing happened with my weight. In fact, I gained some back. Then my Body Circuit hit me over the head and I zapped it, and the weight started to come off. My body is like a weight-loss machine. I'm less hungry, more excited about my life, and so proud that I am losing weight. When Laurel used the term "the joy of weight loss" I didn't think it would happen to me. It HAPPENED!

The Joy of Weight Loss Checklist

☐ I will never judge myself for my weight.

☐ I will only release weight out of self-love.

☐ I will release weight at a rate that is perfect for me – not more or less.

☐ If I do not have the joy of weight loss, I will clear away more circuits.

☐ I will create a vibrant home environment, throwing out most Stress Foods.

☐ I will only wear clothes that enhance my body pride.

☐ I will say this: "No thanks. I am not hungry. I do not eat unless I am hungry."

☐ I will try out the EBT 3-Point Eating Plan: eat only when hungry, eat healthy, take a 12-hour food rest (14 hours for low set point or high body weight).

☐ I will move in joy twice daily, including 30 minutes of exercise, to enjoy my body and myself.

☐ If my set point is in stress (4 or 5), I will access additional healthcare strategies as needed to lighten my stress load.

☐ I will check with my physician to be sure I am as healthy as can be.

☐ I will take all the medications I need and none that I do not.

☐ I will take a therapeutic vitamin and two grams of fish oil daily.

☐ I will enjoy small amounts of hunger, the sign that I am releasing weight.

☐ I will bring to mind my reward for releasing weight and score a Joy Point.

☐ I will continue my Vibrancy Plan, adjusting it to meet my needs.

☐ I will watch for my body to turn into a "weight releasing" machine.

☐ I will release weight until I have reclaimed my genetic body build.

☐ I will take pride in achieving weight loss that lasts.

☐ I will continue with EBT until I have all seven rewards and am wired at One.

I have stopped being anxious about getting enough food. I used to keep a banana in my purse "just in case" I was hungry. Then it dawned on me that I have plenty of food with me all the time. It's on my body! If I'm a little hungry, then my body automatically takes energy from my belly fat, so I do not need that banana. How liberating!

Celebrate what you have accomplished and continue raising your set point. Check off strategies that appeal to you for releasing extra weight. Use them when the *time is right* and savor the pleasure of discovering the *right weight for you!* Watch your weight comfort zone change as your brain changes. It is fascinating to experience!

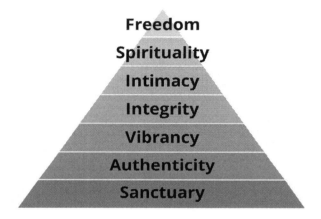

Wired for Joy

Congratulations on completing the Joy Challenge. When you began this challenge, you may have wondered how you could change a neuron in your brain that collaborates with other neurons to trigger you to overeat or repeat other patterns that you do not like. Now you know how to train a neuron as part of a team effort within to make yourself more resilient, and thus happier and healthier.

By using your conscious mind to train your unconscious mind, your brain and your life change. Our genes give us the capacity to remodel our brain based on experience. The brain constantly reorganizes itself, updating our wiring. In the most simply organized way, what you do at each fork in the road depends on the type of circuit that is activated in the moment. Use the Vibrancy Plan and the My Power Grind Ins in this book during the next 30 days to make these changes solid. Then, move right into deepening your rewards, starting with the EBT Kit 1 Sanctuary, and moving through the courses (one for each reward) until you are wired at One. Advanced EBT courses are included with all memberships in the EBT Online Community (ebt.org).

Now you have the power to make changing your brain simpler and more efficient, fun, and exciting to do. The reptilian brain still isn't happy you are doing this, so I invite you to join with others in our mutual goal of outsmarting the reptile within, moving up our set point and living a life in which more of our dreams really *do* come true.

Acknowledgments

This quick course in EBT was 10 years in the writing, as it took piecing together a string of advances in the method to make it possible. The initial impetus for the work came in 2010 with the publication of *Wired for Joy*, which explained the early version of the EBT 5-Point System and reflected my enthusiasm for having discovered the five brain states, not the least of which was unbridled joy.

Late in the writing of that book, new findings in emotional plasticity were forthcoming from New York University, findings that led to the awareness that rewiring the circuits in the brain's "5th Drawer" held the most opportunity for personal transformation.

We reassembled the program to align with this emerging neuroscience and made it simpler, easier, and more fun to use. Meanwhile, technology began taking over healthcare, and my son, Joe Mellin, a business designer, developed a platform for remote EBT services, and helped us see that an online hub of support could provide global access to the tools. He designed an online "emotional gym" for EBT that brought people together to learn the tools solo or to connect in small groups. Dev Singh, now our Chief Technology Officer, and Andrea Singh, EBT's Senior Software Engineer, have developed that state-of-the-art platform over the last six years, bringing their own sensibilities to the design. I am grateful for their creativity, skill, and dedication.

I am thankful for Michael McClure, Director of Member Support, who has contributed to EBT leadership, marketing, and communications for more than eight years, attending to member needs and juggling his many roles with precision and grace. Kelly McGrath has coordinated the method's infrastructure for nearly 20 years and has offered her steadfast support during this transition. Walt Rose led the way in simplifying the method as scalable healthcare, in which members could learn the tools, and potentially avoid excessive reliance on medications, medical procedures, and devices. The empowering nature of the online community appealed to Walt, as he saw it was "people helping people help themselves" to move forward in life.

Early in my work, a colleague, Lee Ann Slinkard, advised me not to write another book until I couldn't stand NOT to write it because there was so much that needed to be shared. We reached that point two years ago, but it took a year to fathom how we could put the entire basic 30-day program into a book. Jill Marsal guided me through writing the proposal, and Colleen Mauro, editor, magazine publisher, and author of *Spiritual Telepathy*, and publishing consultant Eileen Duhné supported our progress in launching this book. Three talented and dedicated editors collaborated on the process of transitioning this course into a book. Frannie Wilson spearheaded the proofing of this publication and brought a fresh eye to the work, and caught me when I explained too much (or too little). She has been tireless in improving the quality of the text and graphics. Michele Welling, MD edited the work, often well into the wee hours of the morning, bringing her medical background to her edits. Jamie Holecek supplied her InDesign and project management experience to the production, and juggled roles to proof and review the instructional design with remarkable dedication. Jami Spittler (Jamison Design), our graphic designer for two decades, provided the cover and interior designs and consulted on the graphics production for this work. As her priorities changed, she helped smooth the transition to our new designer, Steven Isakson, who brought his unique talents to the project. Without each of them, this book would not have been created.

The "pioneers of EBT" for this book and my related book on stress overload include outstanding researchers, each with a body of work that has contributed to the development of the method. The leadership of Charles E. Irwin, Jr., MD in interdisciplinary adolescent health training formed the foundation for the EBT method. Without his dedication to adolescent health, EBT would never have been launched. The core circle of researchers include: Igor Mitrovic, MD, Michael Merzenich, PhD, Lynda Frassetto, MD, Lindsey Fish, MD, Elizabeth Phelps, PhD, Joseph LeDoux, PhD, Bruce McEwen, PhD, Mary Dallman, PhD, Elissa Epel, PhD, Robert Lustig, MD, John Foreyt, PhD, and Nancy Adler, PhD. Without their research and dedication, there would be no EBT.

I am particularly grateful to Patricia Robertson, MD, Sue Carlisle, MD, PhD, Carol Miller, MD, Lori Karan, MD, Kari Connelly, MD, Tracy Fulton, PhD, Melissa Kerr, PhD, Anna Spielvogel, MD, Kim Mulvihill, MD, and Amy Levine, EdD as each has contributed fresh ideas and support for this method at critical junctures in its development. Many EBT clinical leaders have made substantial contributions to this work, including Judy Zehr, LPC, our Director of Community Education, who integrated attachment theory into the conceptual basis of the method, and Michele Welling, MD, who brought her medical perspectives on addiction to EBT, and directs professional certification training. Arinn Testa, PsyD shepherds the method through research planning. Early on, she participated as a trainer in an NIH study on EBT. Mary Croughan, PhD offered guidance about the development of EBT well after her days of analyzing the method's research data had passed. Marion Nestle, PhD, supported the work early on in its transition from pediatrics to family medicine. Dede Taylor advised us through one of our most vulnerable periods and developed our interest in work-site coaching and seminars in EBT. I am grateful to each of them for their generous contributions. I am grateful to Kevin Grumbach, MD, Chair of Family and Community Medicine, and Sam Hawgood, MD, Chancellor, both of UCSF, for their support of the method. Mary Charlson, MD, and Janey Peterson, EdD, of the Center for Complementary and Integrative Medicine, Weill Cornell Medical College advised me on the application of EBT to heart disease and pregnancy research and Kelly Webber, PhD conducted research on the method at the University of Kentucky. Paula Ernst, Tammy Thorton, Lisa McCoy, and Molly Harding were instrumental in supporting an EBT obesity study in association with the public health department in Hagerstown, Maryland.

Many EBT Trainers have contributed to the development of this book, delivering the program and then making important recommendations that have improved its content and process. They include: David Ingebritsen, PhD, LPC, Barbara Gabriel, LPC, Eve Lowry, RD, Denice Keepin, LPC, Deanne Hamilton, MS, RD, Robin Anderson, RD, Micheline Vargas, DrPH, Bonnie Hoag, LPC, Bill Mory, LPC, Sylvia Cramer, DrPH, Carra Richling, RD, and Molly Reno, JD. The memory of psychologist Anne Brown, PhD still influences my thinking about the method.

Special thanks to Seth Kester-Irwin, Nancie Kester, and Charles Irwin for their love and support. Priscilla Christopher, Emily Kearney, Jock Begg, Pamela Steckroat, Janice and Ralph Echenique, Dan Rosenthal, Saunterre Irish, Meghan Decker, Anna O'Connor, Diana Hurlbut, Leah Nafius, Martha Lupe, Sean Foy, Martha Shumway, Tommy Odetto, and Bob Crowder have given to the work in unique and meaningful ways. I am grateful to Lynn and Bruce McDermott, Gail and Bill Hutchinson, Catherine and Dick Krell, Peggy and Jim Galbraith, Jack Grehan, Kela and Carlos Cabrales, Mike Mooney, Skye Reese, and Susie Mooney, Nancy and Jamey Saunders, Jim and Lili

King, Tatihana and George Morales, Justine and Bruce Fairey, Marcia and David Sperling, Keith Chamberlin, Jon Donovan, Brian Strunk, Samantha Wechsler, Lynne Anderson, and Kathleen Wilson for their support during the writing of this book. Beth Tabakin's insights were instrumental to our success during this time of transition. Beth Pawlick has inspired me with her kindness and care. I am very grateful to our exceptional accountant David Bott for his dedication to EBT, and to our business attorney, Bryant Young, and to our intellectual property attorneys Larry Townsend and Steven Nielsen for their crucial advice over the years. Bob Mellin and Sharon Nielsen were instrumental in the early development of EBT when it focused on the treatment of pediatric obesity and its transition into brain training to promote optimal well-being in adults. I am very grateful to them for believing in the method, and helping so many children and families learn the skills. Without their support, there would be no EBT.

My deepest thanks go to my family. My son John and his wife Anastasia's influences have been woven into this book, as both John's understandings from literature and philosophy, and his astute edits of this work have strengthened it considerably. Ana, a pharmacist, is a strong advocate for deriving one's "chemicals" naturally through food ("nutritional power") and a healthy lifestyle rather than from medications. Their son, Henry John, was born just as this book went to press, and already lights up my life. My son Joe and his fiancée Megan share their passions for personal growth as well as systems design and technology with me. Their shared joie de vivre is catching! Megan has brought her Kansas values into our family and enriched us all. My daughter Haley has been a model for me of moving forward authentically in life, and of having sensitivity for animals, teaching me to guide spiders out of the house rather than killing them. She and Joe are now helping people become conservationists, preserving their own acre of land in Oregon or Guatemala to support biodiversity. Still, after more than 40 years, I cherish the memory of my first child, Riley.

When my partner Walt and I met five years ago, he did not fully appreciate the challenges of being with a woman who was in love with EBT. However, soon he shared my passion and became a driving force behind making EBT into scalable emotional healthcare. During these years, Walt has had plenty of "moments of opportunity" to use the stress tools, and, as a result, this book is his accomplishment as much as it is mine. Walt's family, Pete and Erin Rose and their children Paige and Gwen, have become family to me, and bring the fun of making "carrot soup" together and a willingness to be there for one another and share our lives. Walt's son Tom and his wife Caroline and their children Ellie and Tommy have touched me with their commitment to family by moving from Pasadena to Texas as Caroline recovered from a serious health issue. She is now using her experience of recovery in writing her own book and giving City of Hope talks to inspire others.

My father, Jack McClure, passed away peacefully during the writing of this work and showed me how to be brave and live out one's natural life, even when doing so is very hard. The McClure family, my brother Steve and his wife Vivian, Michael and Colleen, Sarah and Ethan, and Lisa have joined my family in continuing the McClure family traditions. My mother, Rosie ("Mackey"), who passed away nine years before my father, and he would be proud of the way their values of taking care of your health, working hard, and loving others now guide all six of their grandchildren.

With the publication of this book and its compatriot book on stress overload, the basic tools of EBT are finally widely available. For the first time in the four decades of developing this method, I can now ride a bike, gallop a horse, or get on an airplane without worrying that if I passed away, the method could pass away with me. That sounds like freedom to me.

I hope you join our mission of bringing EBT to more people to raise their set point and, over time, each do our small but important part to raise the set point of the planet.

Last, I'm grateful to the many EBT participants who apply the tools with enthusiasm, often arriving at new ways to use them, adding to the effectiveness of the method. Also, as they rewire a circuit or spiral up to One, they radiate joy that is contagious and has inspired me as I created this course. I thank them for allowing me to follow their experiences and to share those learnings with you.

Selected Reading

What follows is a list of researchers whose body of work contributed to the conceptual basis of the method and one or more citations of their research. For each researcher, their recent books published in the popular press have been listed first. Several early studies have been included below to show the history of the method.

Hilde Bruch

Bruch, H. & Touraine, G. (1940). Obesity in childhood: V. The family frame of obese children. *Psychosomatic Medicine* 2:142-206.

Mary Dallman

Dallman, M.F. (2010). Stress-induced obesity and the emotional nervous system. *Trends in Endocrinology and Metabolism* 21:159-165.

Antonio Damasio

Damasio, A. (2003). *Looking for Spinoza: Joy, Sorrow, and the Feeling Brain.* Harcourt, Inc.

Fox, G.R., Kaplan, J., Damasio, H., & Damasio, A. (2015). Neural correlates of gratitude. *Frontiers in Psychology* 6:1491.

Damasio, A. & Carvalho, G.B. (2013) The nature of feelings: Evolutionary and neurobiological origins. *National Review of Neuroscience* 14:143-152.

Richard Davidson

Davidson, R.J. & McEwen, B.S. (2012). Social influences on neuroplasticity: Stress and interventions to promote well-being. *Nature Neuroscience* 15:689-695.

Davidson, R.J. (2008). Spirituality and medicine: Science and practice. *Annals of Family Medicine* 6:388-389.

Davidson, R.J., Jackson, D.C., & Kalin, N.H. (2000). Emotion, plasticity, context, and regulation: Perspectives from affective neuroscience. *Psychological Bulletin* 126:890-909.

Paul Ekman

Dalai Lama, Ekman, P. (2008). *Emotional Awareness: Overcoming the obstacles to psychological balance and compassion*. Times Books.

Sauter, D.A., Eisner, F., Ekman, P., & Scott, S.K. (2010). Cross-cultural recognition of basic emotions through nonverbal emotional vocalizations. *Proceedings of the National Academy of Sciences* 107: 2408-2412.

Ekman, P. (2009). Darwin's contributions to our understanding of emotional expressions. *Philosophical Transactions of The Royal Society of London, Series B, Biological Sciences* 364:3449-3451.

Elissa Epel

Blackburn, E. & Epel, E. (2017). *The Telomere Effect: A Revolutionary Approach to Living Younger, Healthier, Longer*. Grand Central Publishing.

Mason, A.E., Laraia, B., Daubenmier, J., Hecht, F.M., Lustig, R.H., Puterman, E., Adler, N., Dallman, M., Kiernan, M., Gearhardt, A.N., & Epel, E.S. (2015). Putting the breaks on the "drive to eat": Pilot effects of naltrexone and reward based eating on food cravings among obese women. *Eating Behaviors* 19:53-56.

Adam, T.C. & Epel, E.S. (2007). Stress, eating and the reward system. *Physiology & Behavior* 91:449-458.

Epel, E.S., McEwen, B., Seeman, T., Matthews, K., Castellazzo, G., Brownell, K., Bell, J., & Ickovics, J.R. (2000). Stress and body shape: stress-induced cortisol secretion is consistently greater among women with central fat. *Psychosomatic Medicine* 62:623-632.

Leonard Epstein

Epstein L.H., Valoski, A., Wing, R.R., & McCurley, J. (1990). Ten-year follow-up of behavioral, family-based treatment for obese children. *Journal of the American Medical Association* 264:2519-2523.

Epstein, L.H., Wing, R.R., Koeske, R., & Valoski, A. (1987). Long-term effects of family-based treatment of childhood obesity. *Journal of Consulting and Clinical Psychology* 55:91-95.

Vincent Felitti

Felitti, V.J., Jakstis, K., Pepper, V., & Ray, A. (2010). Obesity: Problem, Solution, or Both? *The Permanente Journal* 14:24-30.

Felitti, V.J., Anda, R.F., Nordenberg, D., et al. (1998). Relationship of childhood abuse and household dysfunction to many of the leading causes of death in adults: The Adverse Childhood Experiences (ACE) Study. *American Journal of Preventive Medicine* 14:245-258.

Felitti, V.J. (1993). Childhood sexual abuse, depression, and family dysfunction in adult obese patients – a case control study. *Southern Medical Journal* 86:732-736.

Lynda Frassetto

Frassetto, L.A., Schloetter, M., Mietus-Synder, M., Morris, R.C., Jr., & Sebastian, A. (2009). Metabolic and physiologic improvements from consuming a paleolithic, hunter-gatherer type diet. *European Journal of Clinical Nutrition* 63:947-955.

Tom Insel

Insel, T.R. (2019). Bending the Curve for Mental Health: Technology for a Public Health Approach. *American Journal of Public Health* 109(Suppl 3): S168–S170.

Insel, T.R. (April 2010). Faulty Circuits. *Scientific American* 302:44-52.

Dacher Keltner

Keltner, D. (2009). *Born to Be Good: The Science of a Meaningful Life*. W.W. Norton.

George Koob

Koob, G.F. & Volkow, N.D. (2010). Neurocircuitry of addiction. *Neuropsychopharmacology* 35:217-238.

Koob, G.F. & Le Moal, M. (2008). Addiction and the brain antireward system. *Annual Review of Psychology* 59:29-53.

Joseph LeDoux

LeDoux, J. (2012). Rethinking the emotional brain. *Neuron* 73:653-676.

LeDoux, J. (2012). Evolution of human emotion: A view through fear. *Progress in Brain Research* 195:431-442.

Robert Lustig

Lustig, R.H. (2017). *The Hacking of the American Mind: The Science Behind the Corporate Takeover of our Bodies and Brains*. Avery.

Lustig, R.H. (2012). *Fat Chance: Beating the Odds Against Sugar, Processed Food, Obesity, and Disease*. Hudson Street Press (Penguin).

Mietus-Snyder M.L. & Lustig, R.H. (2008). Childhood obesity: Adrift in the "limbic triangle." *Annual Review of Medicine* 59:147-162.

Bruce McEwen

McEwen, B. (2002). *The End of Stress as We Know It*. Dana Press.

Picard, M. & McEwen, B.S. (2018). Psychological stress and mitochondria: A conceptual framework. *Psychosomatic Medicine* 80:126-140.

McEwen, B.S., & Gianaros, P.J. (2011). Stress- and allostasis-induced brain plasticity. *Annual Review of Medicine* 62:431-445.

Juster, R.P., McEwen, B.S., & Lupien, S.J. (2010). Allostatic load biomarkers of chronic stress and impact on health and cognition. *Neuroscience and Biobehavioral Reviews* 35:2-16.

McEwen, B.S. (2009). The brain is the central organ of stress and adaptation. *NeuroImage* 47:911-913.

Laurel Mellin

Mellin L. (2010). *Wired for Joy: A Revolutionary Method for Creating Happiness from Within.* Hay House, Inc.

Mellin, L. (2013). *Emotional plasticity theory: Preliminary evaluation of changes in stress-related variables in obese adults.* (Northcentral University). ProQuest Dissertations and Theses, 307.

Mellin, L., Croughan, M., & Dickey, L. (1997). The Solution Method: 2-year trends in weight, blood pressure, exercise, depression and functioning of adults trained in developmental skills. *Journal of the American Dietetic Association* 97:1133-1138.

McNutt, S.W., Hu, Y., Schreiber, G.B., Crawford, P.B., Obarzanek, E., & Mellin, L. (1997). A longitudinal study of dietary practices of black and white girls 9 and 10 years old at enrollment: the NHLBI Growth and Health Study. *Journal of Adolescent Health* 20:27-37.

Mellin, L., Irwin, C., & Scully, S. (1992). Prevalence of disordered eating in girls: A survey of middle-class children. *Journal of the American Dietetic Association* 92:851-853.

Mellin, L., Slinkard, L.A., & Irwin, C.E., Jr. (1987). Adolescent obesity intervention: Validation of the SHAPEDOWN program. *Journal of the American Dietetic Association* 87:333-338.

Michael Merzenich

Merzenich, M. (2013). *Soft-Wired: How the New Science of Brain Plasticity Can Change Your Life.* Parnassus Publishing.

Merzenich, M.M., Van Vleet, T.M., & Nahum, M. (2014). Brain plasticity-based therapeutics. *Frontiers in Human Neuroscience* 8:385.

Mahncke, H.W., Connor, B.B., Appleman, J., Ahsanuddin, O.N., Hardy, J.L., Wood, R.A., Joyce, N.M., Boniske, T., Atkins, S.M., & Merzenich, M.M. (2006). Memory enhancement in healthy older adults using a brain plasticity-based training program: A randomized, controlled study. *Proceedings of the National Academy of Science U.S.A.* 103:12523-12528.

Temple, E., Deutsch, G.K., Poldrack, R.A., Miller, S.L., Tallal, P., Merzenich, M.M., & Gabrieli, J.D. (2003). Neural deficits in children with dyslexia ameliorated by behavioral remediation: Evidence from functional MRI. *Proceedings of the National Academy of Science U.S.A.* 100:2860-2865.

Igor Mitrovic

Kurtzman, L. (2014). Neurobiologist Shares Personal Journey, Life Lessons in 'Last Lecture.' *UCSF News*. www.youtube.com/watch?v=uKjvQSBaWKQ

Mitrovic, I., Fish de Peña, L., Frassetto, L.A., & Mellin, L. (2011). Rewiring the stress response: A new paradigm for health care. *Hypothesis* 9:1:e1-e5.

Mitrovic, I., Mellin, L., & Fish de Peña, L. (2008). *Emotional brain training: The neurobiology of brain retraining for promotion of adaptive behaviors and state of well-being.* pp. 1-19. Institute for Health Solutions.

Bruce Perry

Perry, B.D. & Szalavitz, M. (2006). *The Boy Who Was Raised as a Dog: And Other Stories from a Child Psychiatrist's Notebook-What Traumatized Children Can Teach Us About Loss, Love, and Healing.* Basic Books.

Perry, B.D. & Hambrick, E.P. (2008). The neurosequential model of therapeutics. *Reclaiming Children and Youth* 17:38-43.

Perry, B.D. & Pollard, R. (1998). Homeostasis, stress, trauma, and adaptation. A neurodevelopmental view of childhood trauma. *Child & Adolescent Psychiatric Clinics of North America* 7:33-51.

Elizabeth Phelps

Raio, C.M., Orederu, T.A., Palazzolo, L., Shurick, A.A., & Phelps, E.A. (2013). Cognitive emotion regulation fails the stress test. *Proceedings of the Natural Academy of Sciences* 110:15139-15144.

Schiller, D., Monfils, M.H., Raio, C.M., Johnson, D.C., LeDoux, J.E., & Phelps, E.A. (2010). Preventing the return of fear in humans using reconsolidation update mechanisms. *Nature* 463:49-53.

Hartley, C.A. & Phelps, E.A. (2010). Changing fear: The neurocircuitry of emotion regulation. *Neuropsychopharmacology* 35:136-146.

Delgado, M.R., Nearing, K.I., LeDoux, J.E., & Phelps, E.A., (2008). Neural circuitry underlying the regulation of conditioned fear and its relation to extinction. *Neuron* 59:829-838.

Stephen Porges

Porges, S., (2011). *The Polyvagal Theory: Neurophysiological Foundations of Emotions, Attachment, Communication, and Self-regulation*. W.W. Norton.

Porges, S. W. & Furman, S. A. (2011). The early development of the autonomic nervous system provides a neural platform for social behavior: A polyvagal perspective. *Infant and Child Development* 20:106-118.

Alan Schore

Schore, A.N. (2009). Relational trauma and the developing right brain: An interface of psychoanalytic self psychology and neuroscience. *Annals of the New York Academy of Sciences* 1159:189-203.

Schore, A.N. (2005). Back to basics: Attachment, affect regulation, and the developing right brain: Linking developmental neuroscience to pediatrics. *Pediatric Reviews* 26:204-217.

Peter Sterling

Sterling, P. (2014). Homeostasis vs. allostasis: Implications for brain function and mental disorders. *Journal of the American Medical Association Psychiatry* 71: 1192-3.

Sterling, P. (2004). Principles of allostasis: Optimal design, predictive regulation, pathophysiology, and rational therapeutics. In J. Schulkin (Ed.), *Allostasis, Homeostasis, and the Costs of Physiological Adaptation* (pp. 17-64). Cambridge University Press.

Janet Tomiyama

Tomiyama, A.J. (2019). Stress and obesity. *Annual Review of Psychology* 70. doi.org/10.1146/annurev-psych-010418-102936.

George Vaillant

Vaillant, G. (2008). *Spiritual Evolution: How We Are Wired for Faith, Hope, and Love*. Broadway Books.

Kelly Webber

Webber K.H., Mellin L., Mayes L., Mitrovic I., & Saulnier M. (2018). Pilot investigation of 2 nondiet approaches to improve weight and health. *Alternative Therapies in Health and Medicine* 24:16-20.

Webber, K.H., Casey, E.M., Mayes, L., Katsumata, Y., & Mellin, L. (2016). A comparison of a behavioral weight loss program to a stress management program: A pilot randomized controlled trial. *Nutrition* 32:904-909.

Your EBT Experience

The goal of EBT is to raise the brain's set point and become wired for joy. It is part of a larger movement, Brain Based Health. By using simple tools to access the brain's natural pathway from stress to joy, we take charge of our health. To improve your success in using Brain Based Health, select one or more of these support options:

☐ **Join the EBT Online Community**

   Visit ebt.org and receive a 25% discount on the Online Plus membership. Use coupon code stressoverload. With this membership, you will have access to our app, videos, workshops, and forum boards.

☐ **Visit the Brain Based Health Blog**

   For the latest science and news about EBT, visit **brainbasedhealth.org**

☐ **Develop a circle of support**

   The emotional brain craves the sound of the human voice so the tools are far more effective when used with others. We offer a variety of telegroup memberships or one-on-one coaching for convenient, private ways to access that emotional support. Also, share Brain Based health with family members and friends. Children learn these tools quite rapidly. Listen to workshops on our site about how to train children and grandchildren in these tools.

☐ **Learn more about certification (for health professionals)**

   If you are a health professional who would like more information about certification as an EBT Provider to provide EBTConcierge Coaching, weekly telegroups, and daily intensives.

The Stress Eating Solution Program

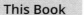

This Book   **+**

The EBT Online Community

- EBT Mobile App for craving relief
- Video demonstrations for each day of the challenge
- More courses: Stress Overload, Advanced EBT & more
- FREE workshops and forum boards
- Coaching and telegroups (additional charge)

This book includes a 25% discount on the Online PLUS membership.
To redeem, visit **EBT.ORG** and enter coupon code: **stresseating**